⁌ The Midwife and the Witch ⁊

Yale University Press
New Haven and London
1966

The Midwife
and the Witch BY THOMAS ROGERS FORBES

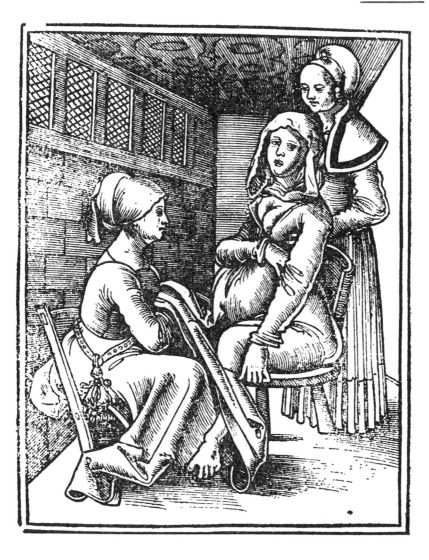

For Helen, Tom, and Bill

⋐§ Preface

Superstition may be briefly and incompletely defined as an unreasoning and unquestioning belief in some aspect of the natural or supernatural. The ideas and practices resulting from such a belief may also be superstitious. Superstitions resemble the people and periods that produced them. They have interest and flavor and variety, and these qualities alone may justify an attempt to collect superstitions. But their fascination has deeper roots. Man has a restless curiosity about the future. Educated or not, he must speculate about coming events, and often his speculation turns to concern about health and safety, the uncertainty of success, fear of what others may think or say or do. His inquisitiveness and uneasiness are never quite subjugated. Superstitions do not often deal with events already past—they are in any case beyond control—or with the split second of the present. They relate instead to the immediate or more distant future, the obscure and shadowed way down which man's steps seem to lie, the path projected in his mind beyond the comforting sunshine of now. He must seek where he can for reassurance that all will be well.

We battle our unrest in various ways. If we are credulous enough, we can take comfort from the protection promised by use of a charm or a superstitious act. The educated man, on the other hand, may be deprived by his very learning of most of his capacity to believe blindly. He must seek a reasoned approach to relieve his fear of the future, and he spurns superstitions, or affects to do so. But let not those who consider themselves enlightened look down on the superstitious. We are all still believers; the difference lies in what we believe, and why.

A superstition is kept alive by credulity, but it nevertheless may once have embodied some logical element. At their genesis some superstitions had an empirical basis or represented correct inferences from false premises. I suspect that if we could discover more about the origin of superstitions we would see more of this. Here, said someone long ago, is a promising way to look into tomorrow or to ward off a threatening turn of events. So he put the method to work. We can assume, too, that his method seemed helpful; otherwise, of course, it would have been abandoned.

Man has always been puzzled by natural phenomena and has always looked for explanations, basing them necessarily on such information as was concurrently available. Thus if we trace chronologically how various people tried to account for a phenomenon, we can glimpse the evolution of knowledge about it. If we begin far enough back, we are likely to find superstitions, and if we continue our review to relatively recent times, we can often discern how rational thought has culminated in a scientific understanding of the problem. We shall also note that an accepted belief of one age may be rejected as nonsense in the next. Truth, after all, is not static but progressive.

Reproductive phenomena have puzzled mankind since very early times. The moment of birth, a climax and a beginning, has ever aroused the imagination; man must always wonder where he came from and how he was produced. These are large questions. The hidden processes of pregnancy, for example, and of the initiation of labor —mysteries still partly unsolved—are not remote but immediate and vital. Each of us has been a participant in these mysteries, and as parents many of us are involved again.

If superstitions can provide a measure of encouragement and reassurance in time of danger, it is not difficult to see why pregnancy and childbirth have been associated with dozens of superstitions. In past centuries both the mother and her infant, unborn and born, were frequently in real danger from disease and malnutrition as well as from ignorant friends and midwives who were able to imperil a normal delivery and incompetent to deal with an emergency. Miscarriage, hemorrhage, infection, and incredible bungling by would-be helpers were all too common, and it was little wonder that an expectant mother sought reassurance from a charm or superstitious observance. Most seem to have been harmless, and many must have owed their long survival to the very real support and encouragement they imparted.

Other obstetrical superstitions, we shall see, purport to supply answers to urgent questions. Can she become pregnant? Is she pregnant? Will it be a boy or girl? Will the baby have a good future? These are questions of impatience. All the riddles will eventually be read, but man does not like to wait, and so he looks for tests to provide the answers now.

Finally we shall consider the role of the midwife in some past centuries. Lowly she may have been, and inept she often was, but it was scarcely her fault. Her not very clean hands guided countless millions of babies into this world; her eventual emancipation from ignorance, incompetence, and poverty and her transformation into today's skillful expert is a chapter of medical history that has been much neglected.

Human reproduction of course is only a part of the broader pattern by which all living beings are maintained. Like other biological processes, reproduction may go astray, resulting in the production of aberrant forms. These irregularities have always puzzled the observer, who sought to explain them as best he could; here again, superstition had to suffice until science provided a better answer. Even the technical vocabulary used to describe normal and abnormal conditions in the reproductive tracts of animals was colored by contemporary knowledge and beliefs. Old ideas about reproduction have left their mark on many words, and we shall look at a few of these too.

I have tried to deal in detail with the topics chosen, but the book as a whole of course is not comprehensive. The material reviewed was selected mostly from the classics and from books, journals, and papers about French, German, and particularly British superstition, folklore, history, and science. All primary sources are indicated, partly in the hope that some readers will wish to make further explorations. Although the bibliography is extensive, it is not intended to be complete. Many excerpts, translated if necessary from original writings, have been included because these passages, usually unfamiliar, add a flavor and immediacy which they themselves can best convey. Punctuation has occasionally been silently modernized to make a meaning clear.

Most of the chapters are based on articles previously published in various journals. Permission to use this material has kindly been granted by the editors and publishers of *The American Journal of Anatomy, The Bulletin of the History of Medicine, The Journal of the History of Medicine and Allied Sciences, Medical History, The Proceedings of the American Philosophical Society,* and *The Yale Journal of Biology and Medicine.* I am also indebted to the Librarians of the Guildhall Library, the Library of the Royal College of Surgeons of England, and the Medical Library, Yale University, for permission to reproduce original pictures and documents in their custody.

Many people have generously helped to make this book possible. Among the medical historians to whom I am particularly indebted for advice and encouragement are Dr. George W. Corner, Dr. Owsei Temkin, the late Dr. John F. Fulton, and Dr. F. N. L. Poynter. Dr. Temkin very kindly read and criticized the manuscript. Dr. Charles Talbot repeatedly guided my steps and also directed me to much of the material in the chapter on word charms. Professor E. Talbot Donaldson, the late Professor G. Lincoln Hendrickson, and the late Dr. Stanley C. Ball gave assistance in technical matters.

Nearly all the research for this book was done in libraries. My debt is great to the librarians and their assistants who at my request brought out the treasures in their care and then suggested other useful books. Miss Madeline E. Stanton, Librarian of the Historical Collections, School of Medicine, Yale University, was gracious and tireless with her help. Mr. Leonard Payne, Librarian of the Royal College of Physicians of London, kindly supplied a number of photostats. Indispensable assistance also was freely given by the staffs of the Historical Library of the Medical School and the Sterling Library at Yale University, the Bodleian Library at Oxford, the Library of the University of Cambridge, and, in London, the libraries of the British Museum, The Folk-Lore Society, the Guildhall, The Institute for Historical Research, Lambeth Palace, The Royal Anthropological Institute, The Royal College of Physicians of London, The Royal College of Surgeons of England, The Royal Society of Medicine, and the Warburg Institute, the Wellcome Historical Medical Library, and the London County Record Office. Dr. E. S. Crelin and Mr. E. V. Newton generously contributed their photographic skills, and Mrs. Inés Cacios searched for books, checked references, and read proof with unfailing care and good nature.

Finally, it is a pleasure to acknowledge the support of this research through grants from the United States Public Health Service (RG 6470), the National Science Foundation (G-8673, G-17597, GS-65), Ciba Pharmaceutical Products, Inc., and the Wellcome Trust.

New Haven, Connecticut   T.R.F.
January 1966

❧ Contents

ᴥ§ Illustrations

The Crowing
Hen

A whistling maid and a crowing hen
Are neither fit for gods nor men.

From time to time over the centuries a farmer has noticed that one of his old hens is taking on the plumage of a rooster and has even begun to crow. Or a hunter has discovered that the "cock" pheasant he killed was actually a female. There was amazement and sometimes consternation as superstitious warnings about crowing hens were remembered. Since the time of Aristotle, such birds, like whistling maids, were considered to be unnatural and to foretell an evil future (Lind, 1963).

> Ill thrives the hapless family that shows
> A cock that's silent and a hen that crows.
> I know not which live more unnatural lives,
> Obeying husbands or commanding wives.
> (Henderson, 1866)

The ancient peoples of many countries killed hens that crowed like cocks. A Westphalian proverb advised,

> Whistling maids and crowing hens
> Should have their necks wrung early.
> (Scheftelowitz, 1913; Jones, 1880)

William Yarrell, a nineteenth-century British biologist (Forbes, 1962) commented (1857):

> Our neighbours and allies the French, who seem to take a wider range in their prejudice against habits which they consider irregular, have the following proverb, which says,

Poule qui change, Prêtre qui danse,
Et Femme qui parle latin,
N'arrivent jamais à belle fin.

(A chicken that crows, a priest who dances,
And a woman who speaks Latin
Are all headed for trouble.)

Numerous related superstitions were widely accepted in many countries. A crowing hen foretold death. The bird could be neither sold nor given away; the unfortunate owner had to eat it. In Bohemia the crowing of a white hen was thought to presage the death of a member of the household, while a similar performance by a red hen predicted a fire, and by a black hen, the visit of a thief. Special protective measures were required to avert evil. A German proverb again recommends punishment for unnatural (i.e. masculine) behavior on the part of a female:

Wenn die Henne kräht vor dem Hahn
Und das Weib redet vor dem Mann
So soll man die Henne braten
Und das Weib mit Prügeln berathen.[1]

(When the hen crows before the cock
And the woman speaks before the man,
Then the hen should be roasted
And the woman beaten with a cudgel.)

Scientists may lack the temerity to explain a whistling maid, but they believe they understand the crowing hen and her occasional aberrant feathered sisters. In most birds, only the left ovary is functional, the right gonad persisting as a rudimentary structure. If the functional left ovary is destroyed by disease (e.g. tuberculosis) or if it atrophies in old age, or if, indeed, it is removed surgically, the rudimentary right testis may begin to grow. This remarkable if belated activity seems to be due to the disappearance of one hormone and the stimulation of another. Development of the rudimentary right ovary appears to be prevented by a female sex hormone (estrogen), which is released by the functional left ovary and is responsible for the appearance and behavior of the normal adult hen. Removal or nonfunction of the left gonad shuts off the supply of estrogen, the female appearance and be-

1. Abbott (1903), Bächtold-Stäubli (1930), Bergen (1899), Dyer (1881), Hopf (1888), Kemp (1935), Wilde (1890).

havior of the bird begin to regress, and the right ovary at last is free to grow. Its development now can be stimulated by another hormone or hormones, in this case released from the pituitary, a key endocrine gland lying under the brain in the center of the head. The normal activity of ovaries and testes is regulated by pituitary hormones. The pituitary, or perhaps the hypothalamus, an adjacent part of the brain, somehow recognizes the disappearance of sex hormone from the blood (the principal means of transport for hormones). The pituitary releases quantities of gonad-stimulating hormones in the effort, so to speak, to restore the situation to normal. In the case of the bird with a nonfunctional left ovary, the rudimentary right ovary is now awakened by the powerful stimulus from the pituitary (van Tienhoven, 1961).

All might be well, and femininity might reign again, if it were not for the curious fact that the newly aroused tissues of the right gonad, though sterile, are largely composed of cells which manufacture androgens or male hormones. The androgens promptly begin to slip into the blood stream and to undertake the task of developing *masculine* structures. Hence the hen gradually acquires a cock's plumage, begins to crow, and pursues other hens. A final complication of this admittedly disturbing situation is that the elderly hen may lose her female qualities rather slowly, even after she has begun to become quite like a male. Then she may go so far as both to crow and to lay a final egg or two. No wonder the villagers shook their heads and the hen's owner considered the chopping block. What did the hen think? Was she a bit confused, or did she cackle inwardly at the prospect of enjoying the best of both worlds, or, henlike, did she simply refuse to contemplate the morrow? We do not know.

Aristotle (384–322 B.C.), as usual, seems to have been the first to record the crowing hen phenomenon, although there is no reason to believe that he was the first to see it. His description of hens that came to look and behave like males is amply supported; his report of the reciprocal assumption by cocks of feminine behavior has doubtful confirmation (Thomson, 1910). In Terence's comedy *Phormio* (161 B.C., IV, 4,706–09), a character enumerating the awesome portents he has seen refers to a crowing hen. Livy, reviewing about 27 B.C. the background of war, tells of numerous strange omens that were observed just before Hannibal's invasion of Italy in 218 B.C.; one such omen was the metamorphosis of a hen into a cock and of a cock into a hen.[2] An

2. *Gallinam in marem, gallum, in feminam sese vertisse* (Livius, 1919 ed.).

epigram (Number 76) of Ausonius (fourth century) mentions the transformation of a peacock into a peahen (White, 1919), and St. Augustine, relating at about the same time the prodigies of antiquity,

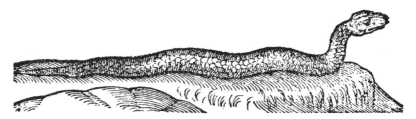

Fig. 1. Basilisk, from Jacob Grevinus, *De venenis*, 1571.

tells how both women and hens were altered to male forms (1610).

Intermingled with these early superstitions was another, already well established before the beginning of the Dark Ages. This was the

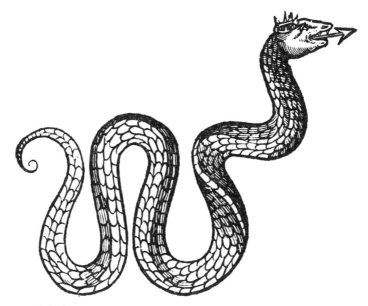

Fig. 2. Basilisk, from Ambroise Paré, *Opera omnia*, 1582. Note the crown.

legend of a small, serpent-like creature known as a *basilisk* (Fig. 1) or *cockatrice,* able to slay with its poisonous breath or even with a glance. Lemnius (1658) quotes the Roman poet Lucan (A.D. 39–65) on the subject. Pliny (A.D. 23–79) said the creature was not over a foot in length, had a crownlike marking on its head (Fig. 2), and killed bushes and shattered rocks by looking or breathing at them.[3] The weasel could kill it but died also in the combat (Rackham, 1947). Aelian's *De natura animalium,* written some time in the third century, adds lurid details: the breath of a basilisk is instantly fatal. Even the snakes (here Aelian quotes Archelaus) feeding on the bodies of dead mules in the African desert retreated into caves or under the sand when the hissing of the cockatrice was heard. Man and beast fled from it for their lives. But, in turn, the basilisk feared the rooster, so that the monster

> is carried away and shakes with terror at sight [of the rooster], and on hearing its crow dies in convulsions. Not ignorant of this fact are they who, travelling through Africa, take along the foster parent [4] of this animal; [the travelers] through fear of the basilisk make the cock a companion on the journey and cherish it as a friend to drive away evil from them. [Gronovius, 1768]

The rooster seems to have been an early and inexpensive form of travel insurance.

Solinus, a contemporary of Aelian, says that the basilisk is found in Cyrene, a city in what is now Libya.

> Africa is on the left of Cyrene and Egypt is on the right, the raging and harborless sea before it, a variety of barbarous nations at its back, an inaccessible solitude which creates the basilisk, a singular evil in the land. This serpent is nearly half a foot in length, the head marked with a small white miter. It is given not only to the destruction of man and other living things but of the land itself, which it defiles and consumes wherever it makes its deadly lair. For it destroys plants, kills trees, even pollutes the winds themselves, so that no flying thing may pass over without infection from a pestilential breath. When it moves, half of its body creeps and the other is upright and lofty. Serpents shudder at its hiss, and hearing it take flight as best they can. Whatever dies from its bite is neither fed on by beasts nor touched by birds. However, it is overcome by weasels, which men thrust into the holes where it lurks. Even then its power is not gone. The inhabitants of Pergamum gave a whole sesterce

3. This is reminiscent of the lethal glances of the legendary Medusa, one of the Gorgons, women with brazen claws and with serpents for hair. Medusa turned to stone all creatures upon whom she gazed. Perseus managed to cut off her head only because he approached while watching her reflection in his polished shield.
4. The basilisk was believed to hatch from a cock's egg; see below.

for the remains of a basilisk so that in the temple of Apollo, distinguished by this warning, spiders would not spin their webs and birds would not fly. [Mommsen, 1864]

Probably in the eleventh century the idea was first set down that the basilisk hatches from a cock's egg. Although this is simply more of the basilisk legend, we must remember the assumption of male plumage by an old hen, sometimes before she has quite finished laying. St. Hildegard (1098–1179), mystic abbess of a Benedictine monastery in Germany, wrote at length about the basilisk. According to her, a toad (which personifies evil) sometimes incubates the egg of a snake or hen. The influence of its body corrupts the developing embryo, and a basilisk emerges. No sooner has it done so than with a great blast the beast tears the earth asunder "even to a depth of five cubits" and hurls itself into the damp ground, remaining there until it reaches maturity. Then the evil creature emerges, ready to destroy all that it sees or breathes upon. Even its dead body pollutes the field or dwelling where it lies (Hildegard, 1855 ed.). Alexander Neckam (1157–1217) may have been the first to suggest that the toad can hatch out a cock's egg.[5] Bartholomew the Englishman, who wrote, probably by 1260, the fascinating *Of the Nature of Things,* adds details to the story of the cockatrice or *regulus* (little king), as it was sometimes known. He says that the dead cockatrice is not harmful and that its ashes are used by the alchemist in the transmutation of metals (Steele, 1893). Vincent of Beauvais, who lived at about the same time as Bartholomew, gives a similar account (Vincentius, 1591).

During the same period Albertus Magnus, Dominican monk and learned natural philosopher, set down additional information. The aged cock lays an egg in a dunghill. The egg has no shell but can resist the strongest blows. The basilisk which is hatched out looks like a cock (Fig. 3), has a snake's tail, and so on. "I don't believe this is true," says Albertus; "nevertheless it is told by Hermes [Trismegistus], alleged author of works on magic and alchemy, and is accepted by many who speak with authority." The great German scholar goes on to comment that "when Hermes teaches that the basilisk is generated in a glass vessel, he does not mean the true basilisk but an alchemical elixir by which metals are transformed."

This brings up a curious confusion. Although one might assume that

5. Armstrong (1958), Robin (1932), Wright (1863).

the live basilisk and the alchemical powder called basilisk were not directly related, a monk called Theophilus or Rugerus in the eleventh or twelfth century told a different tale in his *De diversis artibus seu diversarum schedula*. Spanish gold, he says, is to be made from red copper, powder of basilisk, human blood, and vinegar. The powder of basilisk is made by putting two aged cocks in an underground stone

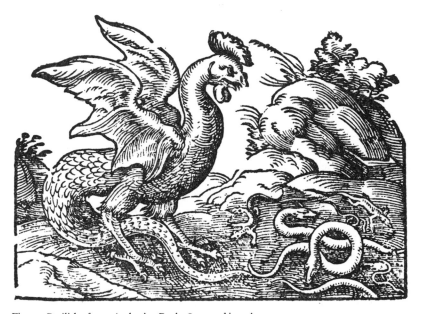

Fig. 3. Basilisk, from Ambroise Paré, *Opera chirurgica,* 1594.

chamber. There must be plenty of food but almost no light. The birds grow fat, mate, and lay eggs. Then the cocks are removed and toads are substituted. The new occupants are fed on bread and incubate the eggs. Baby chicks hatch out, but after a week they grow snakes' tails. Now the stone pavement becomes important, as it keeps the little monsters from burrowing into the earth. They are placed in large, perforated brass vessels, the tops are closed, and the whole affair is buried in the ground for six months. Fine dirt sifts in through the perforations and feeds the basilisks.

At the end of this period, the vessels are taken up and heated over a fire until the contents are consumed. The ashes are pulverized, dried, and mixed with powdered human blood and vinegar. The paste is spread on both sides of very thin sheets of pure red copper, and the sheets are placed in the fire until they become white hot. They are removed, quenched, and again anointed with the mixture. The process is repeated until the copper disappears and is replaced by fine gold (Hendrie, 1847; Thorndike, 1923).

The basilisk legend seems to have reached full bloom in the sixteenth century.[6] As the stories were retold, they were of course improved on and embellished until there was achieved a fairly clear picture of the imaginary beast. Imaginary to us, that is; it must be remembered that for centuries the layman fully accepted the chilling superstition of the basilisks, and many scholars solemnly debated the details of its origin, life, and wondrous powers. Let us examine a few of the records.

Johannes Cuba's *Hortus sanitatis,* probably written late in the fifteenth century, was delightfully translated about 1521 by L. Andrewe as *The Noble Lyfe and Natures of Man, of Bestes, Serpentys, Fowles & Fisshes.* Of the basilisk it is reported that he is:

> kynge of serpentis / for all other serpētes fle from hym / for wyth hys brethe he sleeth [slayeth] them / also if he se man or woman he sleeth them wᵗ [with] his sight / there may no birde passe by hym they must nedys dye. . . . where it cōmeth it brēneth all yᵉ grasse up save only aboute his hole or denne there it is nat bront [burnt]. Some say yᵗ [that] he cōmeth of a cockes egge for whan a cocke becometh olde than he layeth an egge without any shale but it hath a skine that is very toughe / but thys egge muste laye in warme doūge [dung] for there it shold lay warme and than be lentgh [length] of tyme ther sholde come a cheken of it and that sholde have a tayle lyke an adder / and that other parte of the body like the cocke. Some say that a serpent or tode bredeth out this egge but therof is no certentye but it is red in old bokes that it cōmeth of a cockis egge. This serpent is overcōmen by yᵉ wesell which is a litell beste. yet yᵉ basiliscus ronneth away from hȳ & the wesell persecuteth hȳ to deth & sleeth him.

6. The accounts published in the sixteenth and seventeenth centuries are too numerous for our complete consideration. Readers seeking further details and references should consult such excellent reviews as those of Kirchmayer (Goldsmid, 1886), Robin (1932), Schultz (Bonetus, 1687), Seligmann (1910, 1922), Thorndike (1960), and Topsel (1658).

Lemnius, already referred to, says that the cock's egg, laid in the dog days of summer, is sometimes yellow and sometimes bluish. He comments,

> The common people of all Europe believe that the basilisk is hatched from a cock's egg and is incubated by a toad; whether this is fable or a true account I cannot say. But in my experience the cock itself hatches out [the basilisk]. In Zeeland, in the town of Zirczeeben in recent times, two old cocks laid eggs and numerous blows could scarcely prevent them from brooding on the eggs. Since the [owner] believed that a basilisk must be hatched therefrom, as he had seen that the cocks wished to sit on their eggs, he crushed the eggs and strangled the cocks.

Lemnius (1658) believed that the basilisk was produced by a kind of spontaneous generation from evil humors accumulated within the cock's body into an egg. Edward Topsel's *The History of Four-Footed Beasts and Serpents* (1658), based chiefly on Conrad Gesner's *Historia animalium* and his posthumous book on serpents, both dating from the previous century, paraphrases Lemnius on the origin of the basilisk. Hieronymus Fabricius (1537–1619), a careful embryologist, tells about the *centeninum,* the small egg popularly believed to be the one hundredth and last laid by a very old hen (Harvey, 1653). He says that this egg lacks a yolk but has albumin, membranes, and shell (Adelmann, 1942). Subsequent tradition was to confuse the *centeninum* with the cock's egg, and as late as the nineteenth century there was a Yorkshire tradition that it is dangerous to eat a "cock's egg," the last small egg a hen lays. Such eggs were carefully blown and the contents were destroyed (Blakeborough, 1898). Giovanni Battista della Porta (1536–1615), a shrewd and fascinating Neapolitan inventor, optician, botanist, magician, author, and cryptographer, said, perhaps with tongue in cheek, that a basilisk-like creature could be produced by soaking a fertile hen's egg in a distillate of "arsenic, serpent's venom, and other evil and pernicious poisons" for several days. Then the egg must be incubated by a hen (Porta, 1910 ed.).

Physical descriptions of the basilisk vary somewhat, but the general concept is of a small creature, part rooster and part snake. "He has a crowned head two spans long and bright red eyes. His color varies between black and yellow" (Lonicerus, 1560). Pictures usually show a cock's head and wings. Encelius describes a kind of subspecies, the forest basilisk or *Haselwurm,* which dwells among the hazel trees (1557). It is rather generally agreed that the sight, breath, and even the flesh are extremely poisonous (Grevinus, 1571; Lovell, 1661). Reginald Scot (1930) makes some attempt to explain the lethal mechanism: "For the poison and disease in the eie infecteth the aire next unto it, and the same proceedeth further, carrying with it the vapor and infection of the corrupted bloud: with the contagion whereof, the eies of the beholders are most apt to be infected."

A basilisk was supposed to have saved a town in Asia besieged by Alexander the Great. The beast glared out from between two stones of the ramparts and killed two hundred Macedonian soldiers on the spot (Chesnel, 1856; Seligman, 1922). Pliny says that when a horseman killed a basilisk with a spear, the venom rose through the weapon and killed not only the rider but the horse (Robin, 1932; Rackham, 1947).

The term cockatrice appears several times in the King James translation of the Old Testament,[7] which was originally written in Hebrew. I am indebted to the late Professor Erwin Goodenough, of Yale University, for his opinion that "There is no indication that the Hebrew writers knew of the cockatrice" and that the two Hebrew words originally translated into English as *cockatrice* are now thought to have meant *serpent.* Shakespeare uses both *cockatrice*[8] and *basilisk,* e.g.,

> Come, basilisk,
> And kill the innocent gazer with thy sight.
> (*2 Henry VI,* III.2.52)[9]

And Edmund Spenser knew the legend:

> Like as the basilisk, of serpent's seed,
> From powerful eyes close venom doth convey
> Into the looker's heart, and killeth far away.
> (*Faerie Queene,* IV.8,39)

Although doubters began to raise questions, belief in the basilisk continued. Ambroise Paré (1510–90), for example, a hard-bitten and realistic surgeon, summarized with apparent credulity the tales of the

7. Prov. 23:32 (see translator's note); Isa. 11:8, 14:29 and 59:5; Jer. 8:17. Also see Armstrong (1958), Robin (1932).
8. *Twelfth Night,* III.4.215; *Richard III,* IV.1.55; *Romeo and Juliet,* III.2.47.
9. Also 2 *Henry VI,* III.2.324; 3 *Henry VI,* III.2.187; *Richard III,* I.2.151; *Cymbeline,* II.4.107; *Winter's Tale,* I.2.388.

ancients about the basilisk (Johnson, 1665). Edward Topsel (1658) states:

> *Galen* among the Physitians only, doubteth whether there be a Cockatrice or no, whose authority in this case must not be followed, seeing it was never given to mortal man to see and know everything, for besides the holy Scriptures unavoidable authority, which both in the prophesie of *Esay* and *Jeremy,* maketh mention of the Cockatrice and her egges: there be many grave humane Writers, whose authority is irrefragable, affirming not only that there be Cockatrices, but also that they infect the air, and kill with their sight.

Paracelsus (1493–1541) accepts the basilisk as a cause of the plague (Peuckert, 1942), and William Salmon, author of *The New London Dispensatory,* a century later retells the legend without question. The creature seems to have persisted in European folklore until recently.[10]

On the other hand, the existence of the basilisk was questioned as early as 1571 by Jacobus Grevinus, who asked, not unreasonably, how anyone could look at the beast long enough to learn the details of its appearance and still survive. Leonardus Vairus wondered about the same thing (1589). More detailed arguments against the existence of the basilisk were formulated in the seventeenth century.[11]

The terror inspired by the basilisk superstition comes alive in an entry for the year 1474 from the *Kurtze Bassler Chronick,* a very interesting day-by-day record of events in the Swiss town of Basel, set down by Johann Gross in 1624:

> On Thursday before [St.] Lawrence's [Day] a rooster was burned together with an egg which it had laid. For there was concern that a dragon would come out. The executioner cut the cock open and found three eggs still inside. For . . . it was always believed that in its old age a cock lays an egg from which a basilisk grows, the egg having been hatched in a dung heap by a snake called Coluber. Thus a basilisk is half cock and half snake.

From other records we learn that when the "cock" laid its egg it had been solemnly charged with sorcery and brought to trial. The prosecutor first showed that sorcerers prized a cock's egg above all else as an

10. Delisle (1902), Sébillot (1906), Seligmann (1922), Wuttke (1900).
11. Bausch (1666), Browne (1646), Rollenhagen (1680).

ingredient in magical brews. The cock, he charged further, was an instrument of Satan because it was an agent in the production of the basilisk, which worked widespread evil. The defense admitted this, but said that the laying of the egg was an unpremeditated and involuntary act and hence violated no law. The prosecution, however, cited the incident of the Gadarene swine [12] and secured a conviction on the basis that animals could be entered into by the devil and should then be destroyed. Condemned to death as a creature possessed by Satan, the cock and its egg were burned at the stake with full legal formalities.[13] The statement that the executioner discovered three more eggs in the cock has more recently been questioned (Evans, 1906), but Cole (1927), reviewing the case in connection with a description of instances he himself observed in which masculinized hens laid eggs, points out that Gross's account of a "rooster's" egg was probably quite correct.

An egg-laying cock is said to have been burned at the stake for its offense in Ireland in 1383. The report adds that in the heat of the fire the egg burst open and a serpent-like animal crept out, only to die in the flames (Baring-Gould, 1896).

On 15 March 1672 Dr. Johann Zwinger, a distinguished theologian of Basel, wrote to a physician friend about an old "rooster" which in thirteen days laid ten small eggs. The shells were thick and the yolk was missing. Two learned doctors dissected the rooster but observed nothing unusual. They decided that if the dissection had been done during the egg-laying, something would have been found (Bruhin, 1869). Two years later Dr. Sebastian Scheffer of Frankfurt wrote to a friend about a rooster observed by an ancestor: "In 1471 an old cock laid and brooded on a small egg behind a cask in the courtyard of [Scheffer's] house, called Greifenstein. The shell was filled with unclotted blood, but the yellow or yolk had the appearance of toad eggs" (Bruhin, 1869). Tiedemann lists a number of other cases reported in the seventeenth century (1814).

About the middle of that century there occurred perhaps the first scientific investigation into the problem of "cocks' eggs." One day in Copenhagen it was reported that a rooster had laid an egg in no less a place than the royal castle. Very fortunately there was on hand a distinguished anatomist, Thomas Bartholin, who also happened to be the royal physician. He looked into the matter and subsequently published

12. Matt. 8:28–32.
13. Chambers (1869), Frazer (1919), Hyde (1916).

a report (1654). The egg, he said, was "smaller than a hen's egg but larger than that of a pigeon, rather elongated, with a white, hard shell and the usual clear liquids. All the courtiers agreed with one voice that no other bird in the hen house could have laid the suspect egg."

It was larger and heavier than a real *centeninum*. Since the king permitted no one, probably for his own safety, to examine the egg, Bartholin regretfully reports that he had to rely for its identification as a cock's egg on the statements of others, allegations which must have been as unsatisfactory to the anatomist as they are to us.

However, on 10 April 1651 His Serene Majesty ordered that Bartholin do an autopsy at court on the body of the cock. The anatomist found large testes and thin, slim vasa deferentia, but he could not identify cither a possible site of production of the egg or a route whereby it could be laid, and he was unable to make final, definite conclusions. Nor can we be sure. Perhaps the egg was laid by the "cock" in question and perhaps the bird was a hen which had undergone external masculinization following atrophy of the ovary owing to disease or old age, or perhaps the egg was laid by a normal hen and mistakenly credited to the dissected bird, which in turn, of course, may have been a normal rooster.

Nineteen years later Bartholin reported his attempt, in the month of May, to incubate both normal hens' eggs and a "cock's" egg by placing them in an alembic of heated sand (1673). The hens' eggs, when opened after the incubation period, were found to be sterile. The "cock's" egg contained only a white, unspoiled, gelatin-like mass. Bartholin expressed his doubt that a cock could, as commonly believed, lay eggs. He recalls: "I found little or no ovary in the oviparous cock dissected by me long since in the Royal Palace in the presence of the Most August King Frederick III, as was expected; hens past producing [*effoetae gallinae*] bear eggs of this kind." The investigator, later in his paper, refers to the popular superstition that cocks' eggs if hatched produce serpents. "Thus far," says Bartholin, "we have found nothing of the sort in eggs thought to be those of cocks." This reminds him of a reported incident that must have supplied a nasty shock to a royal chef:

> As to the hen's egg, it is recently recorded that in Florence . . .
> when a platter of eggs was being prepared for the meal of His
> Most Serene Majesty, one egg was broken and was found to con-

tain a snake. One may doubt whether this was a cock's egg; more likely it was the egg of a hen impregnated by a snake.

Science had not yet displaced the superstition, but we must salute this Danish anatomist for his scientific rather than speculative attack on the problem.

In 1710, thirty-seven years after the publication of Bartholin's second report, there appeared in the *Histoire de l'Academie royale des Sciences* a notable paper by Lapeyronie. After urging the importance not only of disclosing new truths but of correcting old errors, he tells how he was able to disprove the twin myths of the cock's egg and the basilisk. A farmer brought Lapeyronie several eggs, smaller than those of a hen, which were claimed positively to have been laid by a young cock. Further, said the farmer, if one of the eggs were incubated a snake would be hatched out, while if the egg were opened immediately it would be seen to contain no yolk but instead a miniature serpent. Lapeyronie opened a number of the eggs in the presence of various dignitaries, and found that in each egg there was indeed no yolk but instead a body which looked like a twisted little snake—a discovery which no doubt delighted the farmer as much as it discomfited the scientist. Lapeyronie then dissected the rooster to which the eggs were credited, thinking it might be a hermaphrodite, but discovered the reproductive organs to be those of a normal male.

Now it was the farmer's turn to be surprised. He had no other rooster, but he continued to find the small eggs. An honest man, he watched his flock, finally identified the bird which was laying the little eggs, and brought her to Lapeyronie. The latter kept the hen for some time, during which she continued to lay. Her new owner noticed that she crowed hoarsely and violently, like a rooster. When she was finally autopsied a hydropic sac, as large as a man's fist and filled with clear fluid, was found. Evidently the sac so painfully obstructed the passage of eggs through the oviduct that the bird writhed and cried out during her effort; her struggles, Lapeyronie believed, were responsible both for the fragmentation and loss of much of the yolk and for the twisting of the chalazae into a serpent-like cord (Lapeyronie, 1710).

About the same time another French naturalist had occasion to confirm the sex of 143 cuckoos, all of the same species, by dissection. Then,

> One day, having killed a completely black one, which I consequently had every reason to consider a male, I was strangely sur-

prised upon opening the body of this bird to find an egg ready for laying. . . . This disconcerted me for a moment, but having reflected that I had noticed in several other birds that the very old females take the plumage of the male, I simply concluded that I had just come on further proof of this. [Levaillant, 1706]

Now this is a very interesting observation. Up to this time the records of spontaneous sex reversal in birds had been concerned with chickens and pheasants. One reason, of course, is that reversal is a relatively rare occurrence. Both chickens and pheasants have been killed for food in great numbers, and thus the likelihood of encountering an instance of sex reversal in a chicken or pheasant was relatively much greater. Also, in both types of fowl the male and female differ conspicuously in appearance and behavior. If cases of sex reversal in such common and numerous birds as the duck were noticed before the eighteenth century, they seem to have gone unrecorded. Obviously reversal can occur in the cuckoo too, as it may in a great many other kinds of birds, but to detect it there must be sexual differences in the plumage, one must also study the internal organs, and a large number of individuals must be examined.

Sex reversal in pheasants was reported several times in the latter half of the eighteenth century. It is interesting that all the birds were in flocks, presumably domesticated, kept by titled individuals. This in turn suggests that the birds were under frequent observation. In England, the Duke of Leeds had a common female pheasant whose plumage became that of the male. The same happened to a golden pheasant belonging to Lady Essex (Edwards, 1764) and to three golden pheasants in the garden of a German prince (Götz, 1780). Buffon, the French naturalist, who reports the British cases, says he was told that the older the female pheasant becomes, the more likely it is that masculinization will occur (Buffon, 1771). Hunters, too, were said to be well aware that five- or six-year-old hen pheasants stop or almost stop laying and gradually acquire male plumage; dissection of such birds confirmed that they were females whose ovaries had atrophied almost to the point of disappearance (Geoffroy Saint-Hilaire, 1841).

A classical report on the pheasant was published by the great British biologist John Hunter, in 1780. He describes three instances of reversal in that bird and one other in Lady Tynte's

favourite pied pea-hen which had produced chickens eight several times; having moulted when about eleven years old, the lady and family were astonished by her [the hen!] displaying the feathers peculiar to the other sex and appeared like a pied peacock. In this process the tail, which became like that of the cock, first made its appearance after moulting; and in the following year, having moulted again, produced similar feathers. In the third year she did the same, and, in addition, had spurs resembling those of a cock.

Hunter also noted a case of reversal in a duck (Fig. 4): "In an old Duck, that had become a Drake in Feather, I often observed that she made a noise like the Drake, and at other times like the Duck as usual" (Forbes, 1965).

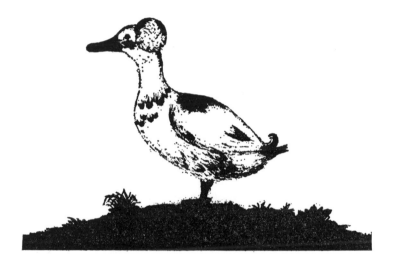

Fig. 4. This sketch of a sex-reversed duck is ascribed to John Hunter. The note is in his handwriting.

Edward Jenner, a famous pupil of Hunter who introduced vaccination as a medical procedure, describes a six-year-old crowing hen that laid a great many tiny eggs and developed a male-type spur on one leg (Jenner, 1931 ed.). The masculinization of old peahens was mentioned again by William Markwick, a naturalist whose comments are appended to those of Gilbert White (1789) in his *Natural History of Selborne*.

In 1788–89 Johann Schneider published an edition of a famous thirteenth-century work on falconry, *De arte venandi cum avibus,* and added some notes and appendices of his own. Butter (1821) quotes one of them, to the effect that old wild female pheasants may develop male plumage; their ovaries are said to be absent or nearly obliterated.

Additional instances of the masculinization of hens and pheasants, and also of ducks, a partridge, a turkey, etc., are reported by Home (1799, 1823), who was John Hunter's brother-in-law, and by Bechstein (1801), Blumenbach (1813), Tiedemann (1814), and Butter. Speaking of reversal in two hens aged thirteen and fifteen years, Butter adds: "Two of my servants, who have lived in farm-houses, inform me, that this change of plumage is by no means uncommon; but that, as soon as it is observed, the hen is immediately killed, because it is looked upon as an omen of ill-luck to any family, where the hens crow" (1821).

Isidore Geoffroy Saint-Hilaire wrote on several occasions about the masculinization of female pheasants, naming three species (*Phasianus colchicus, P. nycthemeros,* and *P. torquatus*) which were observed in captivity.[14] In each instance the bird, after reaching an age of five years or more, stopped laying and then underwent a change in both plumage and voice. The ovaries were atrophic. This author offered the ingenious (even if incorrect) theory that the drabness of female plumage during the sexually active period is due to the fact that the reproductive organs are receiving a special, rich supply of arterial blood; when, in old age, the gonads atrophy and no longer require the "privilege" they had enjoyed, the extra blood is available elsewhere, thus making possible the assumption of masculine form and gay male plumage (Geoffroy Saint-Hilaire, 1822–25, 1841). Several observers pointed out the similarity in certain species of the drab plumage of capon and of normal female. Geoffroy Saint-Hilaire's theory, antedating by twenty-seven years Berthold's classic paper on the endocrine function of the cock's testis (1849; Forbes, 1949), in itself seems significant in the evolution of the idea that the blood supplies something

14. See pp. 19–20 below for equivalent modern scientific names.

necessary for the appearance of secondary sex characters and that, as a corollary, absence of the blood-borne material results in failure of these characters to appear.

Brandt [15] has pointed out that a German anatomist, J. F. Meckel the Younger, in 1824 also attempted a physiological explanation for reversal of plumage when he said that many female birds "when they cease to be fertile, more or less distinctly, now and then, assume male plumage as the formative activity adjusts itself more strongly for the nature of the individual. It would be important to observe, in cases of this kind, whether or not the female coloring again appears." Like Geoffroy Saint-Hilaire, Meckel came creditably close to the mark.

The idea that not only old age but disease may interrupt ovarian function, with consequent masculinization, was perhaps first suggested by the able British biologist William Yarrell. He studied seven hen pheasants having various degrees of male plumage; in every case the ovary was shrunken, purple, and hard, and the oviduct was also pathological. These were not elderly birds. A partridge not more than a year old also possessed partly male feathering and a diseased reproductive system.

Yarrell in 1827 described what seems to have amounted to his ovariectomy of a pheasant, although this procedure is not specified. A piece of oviduct was pulled out through a flank incision and excised; presumably the operation was followed by destruction of the ovary, perhaps through damage to its blood supply, since the bird afterward

> makes an imperfect attempt to imitate the crow of the cock, there is an increase in the size of the comb, and a spur or spurs shoot out, but remain short and blunt. . . . But a more singular point is, the peculiar shape of the lower part of the back in these birds, from the want of that enlargement of the bones, observed in all true females, by which they obtain a breadth of pelvis sufficient to allow a safe passage to the perfect egg.

This scientist apparently was also the first person to seek, by a critical experiment, proof of the thesis that masculinization follows cessation of ovarian function. In addition, he made an astute and early observation on the need for the presence of the ovary if the bony conformation typical of the adult female is to develop. His later reports (1831, 1843,

15. Brandt's review and bibliography are the most extensive I have encountered. The interested reader should consult them for additional cases.

1857) confirm his hypothesis, as do Nilsson's (1845) and Sundevall's (1845, 1854) studies of the heathcock or capercaillie, *Tetrao urogallus,* and blackcock, *T. tetrix.*

In the period from 1836 to 1892 many masculinized female birds were reported. The accounts are, usually, either simple descriptions or observations supplemented by careful anatomical study. The first group includes further cases of masculinization in the common hen.[16] Some of the other birds which were masculinized are listed below. In each case the scientific name is first given as originally cited; in parentheses are the modern equivalent, if different, followed by the common name.[17]

Anas boschas (*A. p. platyrhynchos* Linné) Mallard (Willey, 1892)
Mareca penelope (Linné) European Widgeon (Gurney, 1888)
Anas marila (*Nyroca m. marila* Linné) Scaup (Blyth, 1849)
Anas nigra Lin. (*Oidemia nigra nigra* Linné) *Common Scoter* (Mauduy, 1849)
Mergus serrator (Linné) Red-breasted Merganser (Gurney, 1888)
Tetrao urogallus (Linné) Capercaillie (Fatio, 1868; Nilsson, 1845; Smith, 1866; Stölker, 1875; Sundevall, 1845, 1854)
Tetrao tetrix (*Lyrurus tetrix tetrix* Linné) Blackcock (Bogdanow, 1868; Pelzeln, 1865; Sundevall, 1845, 1854; Tobias, 1854)
Tetrao urogalloides Middend. (probably *T. parvirostris turensis* Buturlin) Siberian Capercaillie (Pelzeln, 1865)
Perdix cinerea Aldrov. (*Perdix p. perdix* Linné) European Partridge (Pelzeln, 1865)
Phasianus nycthemeros (*Genneaus n. nycthemerus* Linné) Silver Pheasant (Geoffroy Saint-Hilaire, 1841)
Phasianus colchicus (*P. c. colchicus* Linné) Caucasian Pheasant (Geoffroy Saint-Hilaire, 1841; Hamilton, 1860; Lorenz, 1887; Pelseln, 1865)
Phasianus mongolicus (*P. phasianus mongolicus* J. F. Brandt) Mongolian Pheasant (Lorenz, 1887)
Phasianus torquatus (*P. colchicus torquatus* Gmelin) Chinese Ringneck Pheasant (Geoffroy Saint-Hilaire, 1841)
Cuculus hepaticus (*C. canorus* Linné) Cuckoo (Payraudeau, 1828)

16. Crisp (1859), Dehn (1856), Green (1836), Homeyer (1868), Jones (1880), Meyer (1866).
17. The late Dr. Stanley C. Ball of the Peabody Museum of Natural History, Yale University, kindly supplied the modern taxonomic nomenclature.

Colaptes mexicanus (*C. cafer collaris* Vigors) Red-shafted Flicker (Cabanis, 1874)

Ruticilla arborea (probably *Lullula arborea arborea* Linné) Wood Lark (Tschusi-Schmidhoffen, 1868, 1875, 1886)

Oriolus chinensis (Linné) (probably *O. diffusus* Sharpe) Oriole (Swinhoe, 1863)

Turdus merula (Linné) Blackbird (Tschusi-Schmidhoffen, 1868)

Ruticilla phoenicurus (*Phoenicurus phoenicurus* Linné) Redstart (Blyth, 1849; Gurney, 1888; Gurney, Jr., 1886; Tschusi-Schmidhoffen, 1886)

"*Blaukehlchen*" (probably *Cyanecula suecica* Linné) Red-spotted Bluethroat (Naumann, 1846)

Lanius collurio (Linné) Red-backed Shrike (Blyth, 1849; Hoy, 1831; Swinhoe, 1863)

Tyranga aestiva (*Pyranga rubra rubra* Linné) Summer Tanager (Audubon, cited by Darwin, 1871)

Loxia chloris (*Chloris chloris* Linné) Greenfinch (Tschusi-Schmidhoffen, 1868)

Pyrrhula vulgaris (*P. europaea* Vieill.) Bullfinch (Cabanis, 1874)

Fringilla coelebs Lin., Chaffinch (Gurney, 1888; Mauduy, 1849)

Linaria (*Acanthis linaria brittanica* Schmied. or *Carduelis flammea* Linné) Redpoll (Blyth, 1849)

Birds not precisely identified (Crisp, 1859; Darwin, 1871; Gurney, 1888; Hamilton, 1862; Koenig-Warthausen, 1854; Larcher, 1873; Leuckart, 1853; Smith, 1859; Sutton, 1885).

This lengthy list could be almost doubled,[18] but it suffices as some indication of the large number of species involved.

The second group of cases is more enlightening. In a hen, for example, with male plumage and spurs, the oviduct was smaller than usual but otherwise normal. There were eggs of various sizes in the ovary, but they contained a viscid colorless liquid instead of yolk. This was an elderly bird that had stopped laying, owing either to age or to a malignant lesion in the stomach; metastasis to the ovary, one suspects, might well have occurred (Eudes-Deslongchamps, 1849). "Melanosis of the ovary from cartilaginous degeneration" was associated with masculinization of hens (Tegetmeier, 1857). In a masculinized bantam hen that died at the age of 13 years, oviposition had ceased five or six years,

18. See, for example, references given by Gurney (1888).

earlier, and male plumage had begun to appear one year before death. The oviduct contained concretions. The ovary was atrophic; "projecting into its upper part was a small tumor about the size of a pea, which sprang from the parts about the upper end of the left kidney and supra-renal capsule." Small encapsulated bodies containing yellow granular material lay loose in the abdominal cavity or were attached to the gizzard or oviduct. The correlation of masculinization with "impairment or complete stoppage of the ovarian function" was emphasized (Turner, 1865). Pathologists' studies of other well-masculinized hens disclosed simple ovarian atrophy (Korschelt, 1888) and an atrophic ovary containing a sarcoma the size of a hazelnut (Stölker, 1875). None of these authors reported the condition of the rudimentary *right* gonad, an unfortunate omission which was probably due to failure to recognize the endocrine activity of this structure.

Toward the end of the nineteenth century an important paper by Brandt appeared; it included by far the most extensive review of the literature that had been published as well as detailed, original observations on a variety of species. The summary of published cases, although not complete, is invaluable. Unfortunately, an adequate elucidation of the embryological basis for adult sexual transformation had not been accomplished at the time his paper was written. His analysis of both masculinization and feminization involved chiefly detailed anatomical descriptions of cases and their arrangement into categories (1889).

Published at about the same time as Brandt's paper were several reports of apparent avian hermaphroditism or pseudohermaphroditism. The latter involves the coexistence in one organism of both male and female accessory and secondary sex characters. In true hermaphroditism, functional ovarian and testicular tissues are also present in the same animal. Sex reversal, on the other hand, constitutes transformation from one sex to the other. It can be appreciated that, particularly when anatomical conditions are not fully described, a dividing line between reversal and hermaphroditism often can be drawn only with difficulty. Three reports will be mentioned as examples.

An eagle had two testes (no histological details), two epididymides, two vasa deferentia, and a well-developed left oviduct. Had these structures been observed fifty years earlier they very probably would have been interpreted as constituting masculinization; Boulart and Chabry (1882), who described the case, believed they were dealing with an instance of hermaphroditism. Now we would consider the bird to be a male showing persistence and development of the left embryonic Müllerian duct.

Another investigator described what appears to have been pseudo-hermaphroditism in four hens and a duck. The hens, although not cock-feathered, crowed like roosters and were large; each had spurs, a male comb, an oviduct, and vasa deferentia. No right gonad could be found. Sections of the "androgynic" ovary revealed no follicles, although a germinal epithelium with primitive germ cells was present, as were medullary cords (a masculine component). The duck's plumage resembled that of a drake. She had an oviduct, an epididymis, and a rete ovarii. No right gonad was seen. The left ovary, when sectioned, appeared rudimentary; it had a well-developed germinal epithelium and medullary tubules. The report lays down the fundamental modern concept of the bisexual foundation that makes sex reversal possible: "every male and every female possess, respectively, female and male characteristics" (Tichomiroff, 1888).

An 1890 description of a chaffinch, *Fringilla coelebs,* if correct, revealed a *rara avis* indeed. In this bird there was the full plumage of a mature male on the right, while on the other side of the midline appeared female plumage. Autopsy showed a left ovary and a right testis. (The gonoducts had been lost in skinning and could not be studied.) Comparison of the gonads with those from a normal male and a normal female convinced the author that he was dealing with a true hermaphrodite, the first avian case, he believed, to have been described (Weber, 1890). Such a bird would now also be called a bilateral gynandromorph—i.e. an individual in which the body appears male on one side and female on the other. The reconciliation of this condition with the concept of endocrine control of secondary sex characters is, of course, extremely difficult, although at least one explanation has been offered (Domm et al., 1934; van Tienhoven, 1961).

Spontaneous avian sex reversal of course continues to be studied in the twentieth century, but we can leave the story here. The crowing hen, feared as a portent of disaster, accused of fathering—or mothering —the basilisk, burned for harboring the devil, suspected of disturbing royalty, perplexing to savant and scientist, has found sanctuary at last in the laboratory.

2

Heifer, Freemartin, and Ridgeling

The great majority of the English words used by biologists and medical men came from Greek and Latin, and usually the derivation of these terms is reasonably clear and undisputed. *Presbyopia,* for example, refers to that annoying condition which most people reach at middle age when longer and longer arms are needed to read the telephone book without glasses. *Presbys* is the Greek word for old man and *ops,* for eye. *Autoclave* is from the Greek word for self and the Latin *clavis,* a key. So an autoclave is literally a self-locking object, as were the earlier models of this important device for the sterilization of surgical instruments and supplies. *Clavicle,* "little key," is the medical name for the collarbone; the word comes from *clavis,* as does *clavichord.* A clavicle has the shape of the S-curved piece of wood or metal used to operate a primitive lock in Roman times, and a clavichord, like some other musical instruments, is played by pressing keys.

A minority of technical words entered the biological and medical vocabularies from nonclassical sources. This is particularly true for terms which describe structures and conditions that have been known for many centuries, names which are used by the layman as well—*heart, hand, ache, sick, calf, seed, plough, fallow, herd.* The derivations of most such words are well established, but there are some others that are fascinating because they are "of uncertain origin," as the dictionary puts it. Here are the stories of three such words.

HEIFER

A heifer, of course, is a young cow; by most definitions, a young cow which has not had a calf. The word *heifer* probably came from Anglo-Saxon and Middle English, but the puzzle is how. Part of the confusion arises because there were or are at least fifty-eight variants of this word, all equivalent to heifer in Anglo-Saxon (Old English), Middle English, and modern English and Scottish dialects.[1]

Heifer and its variants may have been coined to identify a young cow, or to refer to an animal kept or penned in a regular pasture. *Haaf, haft, heaf, heave, heff,* and *heft* are all English and Scottish dialect terms meaning a particular place on a pasture or common where a particular flock of sheep regularly feeds.[2] *Heck* in English dialect meant a pen or enclosure, as does *hoc* in Dutch. But sheep were not called heifers, so possibly the name was used for young cattle grazing with the sheep. *Haft* and *heft* as verbs also meant to restrain or retain. (They are related to Old Saxon *heftian* and German *heften,* make fast, and to Old Norse *hefta,* bind or fetter.[3]) The second syllable, *-fer,* as in *heckfer,* possibly designated a cow or bull (see below) or, at first, any domestic animal kept in an enclosure. A *hafted* or *hefted* cow was one suffering from long retention of milk.

It has also been suggested that there may be significance in the similarity of heifer and its variants to names for some of the other domestic animals. For example, *heafer* and *heafor* were Anglo-Saxon names for a male goat (cf. Icelandic *hafr*), and *hyfr* was an old English term for a spayed goat. *Aver, ever,* and *heaver* were English dialect names for a boar, related to Old English *eofor* and modern German *Eber,* which also mean boar.[4] *Heavier* meant a castrate stag, possibly because such a beast is larger and heavier than the intact animal (Yarrell, 1857; Grant and Murison, 1956) or perhaps because this term was cognate with others already mentioned.

1. *Arger, ayfer, effer, effker, haffer, hafir, haifer, haifir, harfer, hawgher, hayfare, hayfarre, hayfer, hayfre, heafor, heahfor, heahfore,* etc. (Friend and Guralnick, 1951; Gove, 1961; Halliwell, 1847; Murray, 1901; Neilson, 1944; Palmer, 1883; Partridge, 1958; Skeat, 1910; Smith, 1911; Wedgwood, 1872; Weekley, 1921; Wright, 1857, 1902).
    2. Halliwell (1847), Jamieson (1882), Murray (1901), Wright (1857, 1902).
    3. Halliwell (1847), Murray (1901), Wright (1857, 1902).
    4. Bosworth and Toller (1898), Clark Hall and Merritt (1960), Grant and Murison (1956), Johanneson (1956), Murray (1901), Palmer (1883), Pennant (1768), Shipley (1945), Wedgwood (1872), Wright (1902), Yarrell (1857).

In Anglo-Saxon, *heah* meant high. It has been suggested that words like *heahfore* and *heafre* meant a high-stepping or high-bounding animal. By this hypothesis, *heahfore* would signify a high-stepping bovine animal. (*Heahðeor* in Anglo-Saxon meant a deer or stag.) The second half of the compound word *heahfore* has at least two possible explanations. One is that it means ox (see below). The other is that *-fore* is related to Anglo-Saxon *faran*, to go, the root from which has come our word *fare*, to travel, as in *wayfarer* and *farewell* and bus *fare*. Certainly a playful young calf is a "high farer" or "high stepper." [5]

FREEMARTIN

A freemartin is the result of a developmental abnormality in cattle, pigs, and other mammals. The freemartin phenomenon has puzzled farmers and herdsmen since antiquity, but has finally been explained (Lillie, 1917). Infrequently, a cow has twins of opposite sex. Sometimes the blood vessels of such twins become fused long before birth so that the two share a common blood supply during their intrauterine life. It is believed that the testes of the male partner begin pouring male hormone into the blood stream at such an early stage that the developing reproductive system of the female twin is profoundly affected. By the time she is born, her ovaries have been modified into testis-like structures, and she has developed male sex ducts, or vasa deferentia, and epididymides. However, since her mammary glands and external genitalia are almost always of the female type, her transformation is by no means complete. Her size and contour are intermediate between cow and bull. To the farmer, her most important defect is that she is sterile, and therefore of much less value than a normal male or female. She is known as a *freemartin*.

John Hunter probably published the first study of the freemartin (1779). On 5 April 1810 his pupil, Edward Jenner, wrote to the Rev. Dr. Worthington:

> Pray don't part with your *freemartin*. It will be a beautiful animal, and docile and useful in your fields as the ox. I have dissected many; but why this mingling of the sexes should arise under such circumstances eludes all my guesses. I was the first who made the

5. Gove (1961), Murray (1901), Palmer (1883), Partridge (1958), Shipley (1945), Skeat (1910), Smith (1911), Weekley (1921), Wyld (1932).

fact known (some thirty years ago) to Mr. Hunter. [Anon., 1887]

In Hunter's study of the freemartin he remarks (1779):

> The Romans called the bull, taurus; they however talked of taurae in the feminine gender. And Stephens observes, that it was thought the Romans meant by taurae, barren cows, and called them by this name because they did not conceive. He also quotes a passage from Columella, lib.i. cap. 22, "and like the taurae, which occupy the place of fertile cows, should be rejected, or sent away." [6] He likewise quotes Varro, De Re Rustica, lib. ii. cap. 5, "The cow which is barren called taura." [7] From which we may reasonably conjecture that the Romans had not the idea of their production.

Harper's Latin Dictionary (Andrews, 1907) defines *taura* as "a barren, hybrid cow, a free-martin," and Georges' dictionary (1880) gives for *taura*, "eine unfruchtbare Zwitterkuh" (an infertile hermaphrodite cow). The Romans seemed to have understood her bisexual nature: *taurus* means bull, but *taura* is the feminine form. So a *taura* was a "female bull," which summarizes the situation neatly. The passages from Varro and Columella cited by Hunter distinguish *taurae* on the basis of their sterility, but Festus (1699) suggests that the term is applied to sterile cows because they no more bear young than do bulls.

Freemartin as applied to cattle was a term in use by 1681. Lisle's *Husbandry* (1722) spoke of freemartin sheep (Murray, 1901). Beilby's *History of Quadrupeds* (1791) commented that the freemartin is well known to farmers. It is of course probable that the term was popularly employed long before it was used in print. The compounds *free martin-heifer, martin-calf*, and *martin-heifer* have also been used.

The problem of the derivation of freemartin is a dual one. The word martin and its variants seem to have been used by themselves before the combined term came into existence. In England and Scotland martin was also written *marten, mart, maert, mert, marte, marti*, and *martir*. *Mart* had appeared in a document by 1307 (Murray, 1901). Martin had somewhat different meanings in different localities, but the basic sense was cow, ox, spayed heifer, or beef.[8] The medieval ro-

---

6. *Taurae, quae locum foecundarum occupant, ablegendae* (Columella, 1745).
7. *Quae sterilis est vacca, taura appellata* (Varro, 1934 ed.).
8. Ballantyne (1910), Jamieson (1882), Macleod and Dewar (1845), Murray (1901), Neilson (1944), Wright (1857, 1902).

mance of *Sir Tristem* (c. 1220) illustrates the use of *martir* (Palmer, 1883):

> Bestes thai brac and bare;
> In quarters thai hem wrought;
> Martirs as it ware,
> That husbond men had bought
>
> (Fytte First, xlii)

Scottish use of the word is seen in the Acts of James IV in 1489: "That all—*martis, muttoun, poultrie*—that war in the handis of his Progenitoaris and Father—cum to our Souerane Lord, to the honorabill sustentation of his house and nobil estate" (Jamieson, 1882).

Often the term was applied to cattle killed for food on Martinmas, the feast of Saint Martin. It was customary for the Anglo-Saxon to butcher cattle, sheep, and hogs at the time of this festival (11 November) so that the meat could be dried, salted, or smoked for winter provisions. Probably nonbreeding animals, including freemartins, were selected for slaughter. *Mart* also came to mean any meat preserved for winter consumption (Wright, 1902). It has also been suggested that *martin* is derived from Saint Martin's name or that of his day, but there seems to be no real proof that the similarity is more than coincidental.[9] In modern Greek, *marti* signifies a sheep fattened for the festival of San Martino (Palmer, 1883).

Another hypothesis, again without real support, is that the Scottish *martyr* (also *marter, martire, mertir*), to hew down or butcher (Palmer, 1883), is related to the Anglo-Saxon *martyr* (from Greek and Latin *martyr*, a witness) (Neilson, 1944), as used to denote an individual put to death for professing his religion. In early Irish law, *mart* identified cattle taken as an annual rent or tax (Neilson, 1944; Murray, 1901). The Gaelic term could also refer to beef or to a heifer (Jamieson, 1882; Wright, 1902).

There are some interesting possibilities regarding the origin of the prefix free- in freemartin. Two theories have already been suggested, and I should like to propose a third.

The English, and particularly the Scottish words *farrow, ferow, ferrow, farraw, furrow, farra, ferra, ferry, furrow cow,* and *ferry cow* refer variously to a cow that is not with calf, to a barren cow, or to a

9. Anon. (1887), Murray (1901), Neilson (1944), Palmer (1883), Wright (1857, 1902).

cow that is not giving milk.[10] Comparable terms from other languages
are: German *Färse*, Middle Low German and Middle High German
verse, Dutch *vaars* or *vaarkow*, and Danish *vaars*, all meaning cow or
heifer; Flemish *verrekow*, *varwekoe*, or *verweko*, a barren cow; West
Friesian and Westphalian *fear*, Gaelic *fearra*, barren, nonpregnant or
not giving milk, Belgian *vare kow*, a cow that is not giving milk.[11] It
may be assumed that a term signifying a barren cow also implies a cow
that does not give milk. Similarly, Jamieson (1882), speaking of *ferry
cow*, a cow that is not with calf and continues to give milk throughout
the winter, remarks: "I suspect that the phrase is radically the same
with Belg. *vare koe*, a cow that yields no more milk. For although it
seems to signify the very reverse, perhaps the original idea was, that a
cow, that did not carry, would by degrees lose her milk entirely."

On the basis of these terms, signifying either simply a cow or a
heifer or an animal that is not carrying out its normal and desirable
functions of reproduction and lactation, it has several times been suggested that free- is a contraction of *ferry*, *farrow*, etc. and designates
the type of *martin* that can produce neither offspring nor milk
(Anon., 1887; Ballantyne, 1910).

A second hypothesis, suggested by Jamieson (1882), is that the
Scottish *ferow*, not carrying a calf, is related to the Anglo-Saxon *faer*,
empty, void, a reference to the sterility of the freemartin. If this is so,
free- may be a contraction of *ferow*.

A third possibility is that free- may have had its origin in one or
more of the words which, in various languages, signify bull or ox (see
discussion of *heahfore*, above). Thus, in addition to Anglo-Saxon
fearr, *fearh*, or *fear*, a bull, there are German *Farre*, Icelandic *farri*,
Old Friesian *fering*, Dutch, Middle Low and Middle High German
var or *varre*, and Old High German *farr*, all meaning bull or ox.[12] According to this reasoning, freemartin would mean bull-like cow or ox-
like cow, just as taura probably signified female bull. If such was the
case, then it is of course reasonable to assume that at the times these
terms came into use, cattle raisers recognized that the freemartin
possesses some essential characteristics of both sexes.

10. These terms are not to be confused with *farrow*, *ferry*, etc., young pig, litter of
pigs, derived from the Anglo-Saxon *fearh* (Kurath and Kuhn, 1959; Murray, 1901;
Skeat, 1910; Wright, 1857).
11. Craigie (1931), Dwelly (1930), Friend and Guralnick (1951), Grant and Murison
(1956), Holthausen (1934), Jamieson (1882), Murray (1901), Neilson (1944), Palmer
(1883), Prick van Wely (1930), Warrack (1911).
12. Bosworth and Toller (1898), Hall (1931), Holthausen (1934), Smith (1911),
Vigfusson (1874), Weekley (1921).

RIDGELING

This is still another biological term of uncertain derivation; again, clearly, it did not come from Latin and Greek (Neilson, 1944). The word has been applied to various domestic animals; most commonly it refers to a male which has been "half castrated," i.e. has had only one testis removed, the other gonad being cryptorchid and relatively inaccessible to the operator. For reasons to be explained, such animals are useless.

Normally, the mammalian testis, which develops embryologically near the kidney, descends toward the end of fetal life or in the first year after birth (depending on the kind of animal) into the pelvis, leaves the body cavity via the inguinal canal, and comes to rest in the scrotum. In cryptorchidism, a not uncommon condition, the testis does not complete this journey, and may not even enter the inguinal canal.[13] It remains instead within the abdominal cavity or within the canal. To remove the gland successfully from either site requires a good deal of surgical skill, much more than is needed for a simple castration. Also, there is increased risk of serious infection. Probably these are the reasons why the removal of cryptorchid testes seems not to have been attempted until the development of modern veterinary surgery.[14]

The ridgeling horse or sheep or dog, having lost his normal testis but retaining an abnormally located gonad, develops atypically. He is sterile, for cryptorchid testes seldom if ever produce sperm; hence he is worthless for breeding. He develops the sex drive of the uncastrated adult male, since the cryptorchid testis retains at least some of its endocrine function. The ridgeling may become unmanageable or even vicious,[15] partly because cryptorchidism may be painful (DeVita, 1953).

> The adult cryptorchid horse is ceaselessly tormented by the sexual instinct. Like the normal stallion, he seeks out the mare and rushes neighing to her. Usually he is not vicious in the usual sense of the word, but when he scents the female, he is soon the victim of "sexual madness." Spirited, indifferent to threats, insensible to blows, completely intractable, he escapes from his handler or breaks his

---

13. John Hunter commented, "it is a very common circumstance, that many quadrupeds have only one testicle in the scrotum; and in such as are killed for food, and from that circumstance come more particularly under observation . . . , we in general find the other testicle in the cavity of the abdomen" (1792).

14. Best (1857), Cadiot (1893), Lush et al. (1930), O'Connor (1931).

15. Hobday (1903), Lush et al. (1930), Miller and West (1953), Williams (1921).

halter. He bites, runs, lashes out with his hoofs, and can seriously injure animals or people nearby, particularly if one attempts to prevent the gratification of his imperious desire. [Cadiot, 1893]

Less frequently, the term ridgeling and its variants described a cryptorchid animal which had not been castrated.[16] Such beasts were also of little or no value; if unilaterally cryptorchid, they were fertile but were not bred, as it was feared that the abnormal condition might be inherited (Williams, 1921); animals retaining both testes in the abdomen or inguinal canals were sterile anyway. In either event, the behavior would not be that of the docile castrate but that of the aggressive, intact male, and the animal might be savage as well.[17] Small wonder that the unfortunate ridgeling was very unpopular indeed.

The *Sporting Magazine* for 1811 reported an "Interesting Horse Cause," or lawsuit, brought to recover the price paid for a horse which, although it had been sold as a gelding, could not be pastured with mares. It developed that this animal was a ridgeling and that two attempts had been made to remove the cryptorchid gonad (Anon., 1811).

Cryptorchidism is said to be more common in Angora goats (approximately 5.5 per cent) than in any other domestic animal (Asdell, 1946; Lush et al., 1930). Mention of a ridgeling goat was the basis of an instance of apparent plagiarism. Idyll III of Theocritus (third century B.C.) includes a reference to a goat: "and beware of the yellow Libyan he goat lest he butt thee with his horns." As the Greek was translated by Zamagna in 1792 into Latin, the lines become *Namque caper Libycus cornu ferit ille, caveto,* "Beware the Libyan goat, for he bears horns" (Zamagna, 1792). Now a passage in the eleventh *Eclogue* of Virgil (70–19 B.C.) is similar to Theocritus' original; Virgil's *occursare capro (cornu ferit ille) caveto* (Ribbeck, 1894) would seem to have influenced Zamagna's much later translation (1792). To make matters more complicated, Thomas Creech (1659–1700), in translating this passage from Theocritus (1713 ed.), and John Dryden (1631–1700), in translating the corresponding passage from Virgil (1887 ed.), wrote almost identical lines—"But 'ware the Libyan Ridgling's butting Head." "And 'ware the Libyan ridgil's butting head" —which were also very free translations. One is glad to report that later scholars were more accurate (Hallard, 1894; Polwhele, 1792).

Canine ridgelings were recorded at least as early as 1702 (Kurath

16. Hunter (1779), Miller and West (1953), Neilson (1944), Wright (1902).
17. Hobday (1903), Lush et al. (1930), O'Connor (1931).

and Kuhn, 1959). The ridgeling boar is called in German dialect *Rig* or *Rigel* (Heyse, 1842; Neilson, 1944). Because its testes retain their endocrine function, the animal's meat, like that of a normal adult male, becomes too strong for human consumption. Since, in addition, the ridgeling boar is sterile and cannot be bred, he is almost worthless (Williams, 1921)

An incompletely caponized fowl was known in Austria as a *Rigler* or *Halbhahn*.[18] The similarity of the former term to *Rig* and *Rigel* is undoubtedly related to the fact that in the half-caponized fowl, as in the ridgeling boar, one testis is left in the abdomen, although for different reasons. John Hunter referred to a cryptorchid bull as a *ridgill* (1779). Variants of ridgeling were even applied loosely to men—e.g. "redgelinges, or guelte [gelded] men" (Boemus, 1555). "I hate a base cowardly Drone, / Worse than a Rigil with one Stone" (Cotton, 1670).

Ridgeling sheep were trouble-makers in any flock. One British community in 1597 had a law barring such animals from the common grazing ground:

> Item a payne [penalty] sett that no personne or personnes shall put any *ridgell tupp* [ridgeling sheep] upon the moore between the feast of St. Luke the Evangelist [18 October] and the natyvitie of *our* Lord god upon payne for every ridgell so found xijd [twelve pence.]

By 1621 the restricted period had been extended:

> A payne sett that no person or persons shall putt any ridgell tupp haveing either butt one or no stone in the codd to the moore or common betwixt Michaelmas [29 September] and Christmas upon payne of everie seuerall offence to forfeit xijd.

The law was still on the books in 1751. The fine had greatly increased, and the restricted period was still longer:

> A pain set that any person or persons that shall keep any ridgell or close tupp [see below] upon the moor or common from the first day of September untill the last day of December each person for each offense three shillings and four pence. [Addy, 1888]

During the 1640s Henry Best, a Yorkshire farmer, kept careful records of his farming activities. Best, who clearly was an educated man,

18. Heinsius (1820), Heyse (1842), Neilson (1944).

begins his journal with a discussion of sheep. He defines normal males (1857 ed.) and then moves on to cryptorchidism:

> Hunge tuppes are such as have both stones in the codde, and these only are to be kept for breeders; because of the experienced adage, omne animal generat sibi simile [every animal produces its own kind]. Close tuppes are such as have both the stones in the ridge of the backe, and are therefor very difficult to geld. Riggon tuppes are such as have one stone in the codde, and the other in the ridge of the back, and therefore the most dainger and difficultie is in geldinge of these, beinge to be cutt in two places before they can be made clean weathers.

Classical descriptions of the ridgeling condition, particularly as it occurred in sheep and cattle, form the basis for one supposed derivation of ridgeling. Marcus Terentius Varro (116–27? B.C.) in his *De re rustica* advised the herdsman that periodically the herd must be examined and counted and that it should be decided how many worthless animals should be removed.[19] Cattle which are useless should be eliminated [20] to make a place for animals of value (Lewis and Short, 1907; Varro, 1934 ed.). Nonius Marcellus, the classical grammarian, lists *reicula,* but applies it to "sheep culled out, whether for age or serious sickness." [21] Samuel Johnson (1805) and numerous other eighteenth- and nineteenth-century lexicographers believed that ridgeling is derived from *rejicula* or *reicula.*[22] There is something to be said for this opinion; the first syllables are similarly pronounced, and both end in a diminutive (*-ling, -ulus*). I have found no evidence, however, that *reicula* referred specifically to a ridgeling, although the herdsman would certainly wish to remove ridgeling sheep or cattle from his flock. Another reason for doubting that ridgeling came from the Latin *reicula* is that the latter term appears to have no direct descendant among the Romance languages.

Several authorities agree that ridgeling and at least some of its variants [23] are apparently derived from ridge, an old term for the spine or

19. *Quot reiculae sint alienandae* (Varro, 1934 ed.).
20. *Reiculae reiciundae.*
21. *Reiculas oves, aut aetate aut morbo graves* (Nonius Marcellus, 1895 ed.).
22. Bailey (1802), Barclay (1799), Fenning (1775), Freund (1840), Perry (1805).
23. Variants of ridgeling include: *redgelinge, reggil, ridgel, ridgelin, ridgell, ridger, ridgil, ridgill, ridgillon, ridgiour, ridgit, ridgul, rig, rigel, rigeld, rigele, rigell, rigelle, riggald, riggelt, riggil, riggilt, rigg'lt, riggold, riggon, riggot, rigil, riglan, rigland, riglin,*

back, close to which the cryptorchid testis was thought to remain.[24] Certainly in the sheep and goat the cryptorchid testis is said to lie near the spine and the kidneys; this is where the fetal gonad normally develops prior to its migration into the pelvis. Henry Best in 1641 (see above) spoke of "Riggon tuppes," male sheep which "have one stone in the codde, and the other in the ridge of the back." Lush et al. (1930) state that "nearly always" in goats and sheep the cryptorchid testis "remains in its original position high in the abdominal cavity just posterior to the kidneys and slightly ventral to them" (p. 5). Thomas Blount, an early lexicographer, in his *Glossographia: or, A Dictionary Interpreting the Hard Words,* published in 1674, says that a "Ridgil is the male of any beast" which is half castrated; "others add that also to be a Ridgil, whose stones never came down; but lie in his reins [kidneys]" (Blount, 1674).

On the other hand, it is reported that cryptorchid testes in the dog are usually found in or near the inguinal canal (DeVita; Lacroix, 1949). A cryptorchid testis in the horse most frequently lies on the ventral abdominal wall, near the pelvic brim.[25] In seventy-seven horses on which Hobday operated for cryptorchidism, a retained testis was in the abdomen in thirty-nine cases and in the inguinal canal in forty-three (1903).

In summary, then, the idea that ridgeling derived from *rejicula* or *reicula* is tempting but is not supported by modern etymologists. The derivation of ridgeling, ridgel, etc. from the ridge of the back appears correct if these terms were first applied to sheep and goats but seems less appropriate in the case of dogs and horses.

In some parts of the United States a ridge runner is a wild horse which may be seen running on the ridge of a hill (Wentworth, 1944). In West Virginia, Ohio, and Missouri a ridge runner is an undisciplined adolescent or a semicastrated, cryptorchid farm animal. Asked the reason for the name, an old farmer explained, "Because you can't keep it down in the valley with the herd; it's always running up on the ridge."

---

rigling, rigsie, rigwiddie, rogel, rudgel, rudger (Addy, 1888; Anon., 1811; Asdell, 1946; Ash, 1775; Barclay, 1779; Best, 1857; Chope, 1891; Creech, 1713; Dryden, 1887; Farmer and Henley, 1903; Hobday, 1903; Hunter, 1779; Hunter and Morris, 1897; Jamieson, 1882; Marshall, 1873; Murray, 1893; Neilson, 1944; Perry, 17-?; Ray, 1674; Skeat, 1914; Wright, 1857, 1902).

24. Neilson (1944), Murray (1901), Wright (1902).
25. Cadiot (1893), Fleming (1902), O'Connor (1931).

3

Pregnancy and
Fertility Tests

Many are the waies Authors have left
for Women to know whether they
be with Child or not, which happen
true in many Women, but not in all.
(Culpeper, 1653)

Whether a woman has become pregnant and whether she is able to become so have been urgent questions since mankind began to speculate about the future. Many are the procedures by which men and women have tried to make nature reply. Most of the "tests" are very old, and almost all of them are unreliable. Ancient or modern, they exemplify man's search for the answers to important mysteries. We shall consider pregnancy and fertility tests together, partly because a distinction between the two often was not drawn by the earlier authorities; it was simply stated that if the test had a certain result, the woman "will bear." Whether this meant that she had conceived, or simply that she could do so, might not be specified.[1]

Uroscopy, diagnosis by examination of the patient's urine, had been practiced since the early days of Arabian medicine and possibly before. The urine of pregnancy was believed to have special features, particularly if it were stored in a glass container for a few days. One characteristic was the pearly film of *kyesteine* reported to form on the surface. The story of this phenomenon has been well told by Marshall (1948), and will not be repeated here. It appears that the surface layer is a result of the stimulation of bacterial growth by the hormones of pregnancy. Curiously enough, although Avicenna, Hippocrates, and Savonarola, according to Marshall, were aware of the changes occurring in

---

1. I have drawn on many sources for this chapter. Particular assistance has been received from the excellent reviews of Bayon (1939), Dawson (1929), Fasbender (1897), Henriksen (1941), and Iversen (1939).

stored pregnancy urine, the *kyesteine* was not fully described until Nauche published his observations in 1831. A century later, Aschheim and Zondek (1928) devised their test, later widely used, which, although it does not depend on the appearance of the specimen, is based also on an increase of pituitary hormones called gonadotrophins in the urine of early pregnancy.

It should be emphasized that both the Aschheim–Zondek method and other new and even simpler tests have a high degree of accuracy. The modern obstetrician can give a reliable answer to the ancient question.

The late Loren C. MacKinney has called attention (1937) to an amusing tale that illustrates the skill once attributed to the uroscopist. In the tenth century, Notker Balbus was a famous healer priest of St. Gall, Switzerland; he also held a post as physician to a certain Duke Henry. One day the duke played a uroscopic practical joke on his medical advisor. Notker, not taken in,

> craftily let it appear that he was deceived into thinking he was dealing with the urine of Duke Henry. When [the Duke] sent to him the urine of a young woman of his court, Notker said, "Now God has worked a miracle and portent, because whoever heard of a man giving birth from his uterus! For about thirty days from now the Duke will carry in his bosom a son born from his womb." Caught out, [the Duke] blushed, and sent a reward to the man of God, although not lest he [Notker] refuse to treat him medically (for he had assumed this obligation), and the woman, considered a virgin by the doctors of St. Gall, he good naturedly took back into his following. For as had been prognosticated, she gave birth. [Ekkehard]

Uroscopy was a tricky business at best, particularly for those pretending to the diagnosis of pregnancy. Savonarola (1384–1463?) began his ponderous discussion, "Pregnancy urines should be regarded with great solemnity" (1561). A sixteenth-century physician advised:

> Meanwhile, furthermore, girls come with urines and ask the doctor to inspect them. Take notice, while they talk with you, whether they are half laughing, or appear suffused with shame; it is an indication from some women . . . whether it is a matter of a furtive mistress whose menses are deficient and who wishes to know

whether she is pregnant, or of an honest woman for other reasons, or assuredly one whose marriage is being spent in sterility and who desires to know the cause of the sterility. Whatever it may be, you will have acted justly and prudently if you state that you are unwilling and moreover are not obliged publicly to [diagnose] for some one else other than the person whose urine it is. [Castro, 1662]

A scornful contemporary pointed out "that very often these diviners are deceived by being given the urine of a man, whom they say is great with child, which quite properly causes roars of laughter" (Joubert, 1578). John Cotta observed in his *A Short Discoverie of the Unobserved Dangers of Severall Sorts of Ignorant and Vnconsiderate* Practisers of Physicke in England (1612):

Erroneously therfore the common sort imagine, that in the vrine is contained the ample vnderstanding of all things necessary to inform a Physition. . . .

But the violent and forcible importunacie of great and mightie Potentates (who vsually prevaile to abuse great and worthie wits vnto base arts and offices) againe compelled me vpon the same rocke, and my own private profite againe inticed me to thinke it dutie and honestie to make profitable vse of wilfull folly, and with toyes to please these that so much desired toyes. The same Apologie for the exercise of vrinary divination, their owne consciences vnto themselves do make that vse it, but they loath the example, and truth is hatefull because incommodious.

Actually, the inspection of urine to determine whether a woman will have a child is mentioned in the fascinating Berlin medical papyrus (Brugsch, 1863), thought to date from the Nineteenth or Twentieth Dynasty (approximately 1350–1100 B.C.). Turbid or sedimented urine indicated that "she will bear." Avicenna (A.D. 980–1037) spoke of a surface cloud, a yellow iridescent color, a cotton-like mass, and granules as diagnostic signs (Gruner, 1930). The same idea turned up in John of Gaddesden's *Rosa anglica practica medicinae a capite ad pedes*,[2] printed in 1492. More details about the appearance of urine in this pregnancy test were given by physicians of that period and a little later (Bonaciolus, 1563; Castro, 1628), but skepticism was also being expressed, particularly by John Cotta, who condemned this kind of di-

2. *The Practical English Rose of Medicine from Head to Feet.*

agnostic effort by listing it in his book, *A Shorte Discoverie of the Vn-
observed Dangers of several sortes of Ignorant and Vnconsiderate
Practices of Physicke in England.*[3]

The surgeon Cornelius Solingen (1693) stated that Fernelius (presumably this was Jean Fernel, 1497–1558, professor of medicine at
Paris) recommended mixing a suspected urine with wine: "If the
liquid becomes turbid, as though beans had been cooked therein, then
the woman is pregnant." But, as Aschheim (1930) points out, Solingen himself remarked, "That such a thing may be true, I let my geese
believe." The same test was also used in what is now Czechoslovakia
(Hovorka and Kronfeld, 1909).

It is a remarkable fact that several of the pregnancy tests that appear
in the early medical papyri of the Egyptians can be traced with reasonable certainty into Greek and thence to Roman and sixteenth-
century medicine. Dawson (1929, 1934), Iversen (1939), and others
have discussed this progression.[4] In Prescription 199 of the great Berlin
medical papyrus, for example, it is directed that wheat and spelt (a
kind of cereal) be placed in two flasks (Wreszinski, 1909) or cloth
packs (Fasbender, 1897) with dates and sand and be watered daily
with the woman's urine. If the grains sprout, she is pregnant.[5] Iversen,
who offers impressive evidence that several European pregnancy tests
are linked to the early Egyptian papyri, bases his argument on his
translation of the Carlsberg papyrus. He dates this document from the
Twelfth Dynasty (about 2000–1800 B.C.) or even earlier. Part of Prescription III of the Carlsberg papyrus is missing, but Iversen believes
that it agrees with Prescription 199 in the much later Berlin papyrus.

Lüring (1888) has pointed to a parallel passage in Galen:

> Make two little holes containing the urine of a pregnant woman;
> in one throw barley and the other wheat. Then sprinkle with the
> urine and shovel earth on top. If the grains of wheat sprout first,
> she will bear a boy, but if the barley seeds, a girl. [Kühn, 1827]

A Galenic test for fertility is similar (Lüring, 1888): when a couple is
childless, put a lentil into the urine of each. The lentil will sprout in
the urine of the fertile individual, but not in that of the sterile one.

---

3. Cotta (1612), Kräutermann (1730), Schurigius (1731).
4. Chabas (1862), Ebers (1895), Erman (1887), Fasbender (1897), Lüring (1888).
5. Here, as in several other prescriptions, futher directions are given for determining
whether the unborn child is boy or girl. The subject of prenatal prediction of sex will
be dealt with in the next chapter.

Priscian (1597) in the fourth century, and Moschion in the sixth (Lüring, 1888), advised putting barley or lentils in two earthen vessels and watering one with the urine of the husband and the other with that of the wife. Sprouting of the seed would show who was fertile. The test turns up in a fourteenth-Century English medical manuscript [6] and in Antonio Guainerio's *De egritudinibus matricis* (1500), one of the very early printed books on a medical subject. In 1540 appeared *The Byrth of Mankynde* (Rösslin), Richard Jonas' translation of *Eucharius* Rösslin's famous *Der Swangern frawe[n] und hebamme[n] Roszgarten* (1513). This very popular work was the first printed book on midwifery and the first to be devoted entirely to this subject. Rösslin and Jonas gave more details for the test, e.g. to plant the grain in "ii. pottes / such as they set gyly-flowers in / fill them with good earth" and to continue to water the pot with urine daily for eight or ten days, watching to see which seeds would germinate and prove thereby the fertility of the men and women, "but see that there come no other water or rayne on the pottes." Rueff (1554) and Khunrath (1623) also endorsed this method.

The appalling *Dreckapotheke* of Paulini (1714) recommended the test, ascribing it to one Peter Beyer or Bayer, a famous sixteenth-century physician of Florence. Bayer's sources, Iversen believes (1939), were a Greek codex and, probably, Galen. Iversen does not accept Ebers' (1895) theory that the test came into European medical literature via Constantine the African (A.D. 1020–87) and the Salernitan School, although Constantine did describe the test (Constantinus Africanus, 1539). Erman (1887) seems to have been the first to call attention to the repetition in Paulini's *Dreckapotheke* of the method which had originally appeared in the Berlin medical papyrus. Le Page Renouf (1873) had also pointed to the close parallel between the method described in the Berlin papyrus and those in *The Experienced Midwife,* a compilation appearing under the pseudonym of Aristotle (1793). It seems certain that this and other pregnancy and fertility tests can be traced back from eighteenth-century European medical lore to the great medical papyri of early antiquity.

Henriksen (1941) reminds us that recent studies indicate that the hormones present in pregnancy urine may indeed stimulate the germi-

---

6. "Take of eytherys wat*er* and put it in-to sondre vessell; sythen put to eyt*her* barlyche and horssysdong, and whether wessell sporgyth hy*m,* is not bareyn" (Holthausen, 1897).

nation of seeds and the growth of plants. The evidence is controversial but important. In the first place, there are "plant hormones" called auxins which accelerate plant growth and development. The most important auxin seems to be indoleacetic acid. It is possibly ingested in meat and is excreted in human urine.[7] However, I have not found a report that the level of urinary auxins increases during pregnancy.

In the second place, studies have been made of the ability of the steroid sex hormones, which are produced by human beings, to accelerate the sprouting of seeds. Estrogens (ovarian hormones) are excreted in the urine in increased amounts during pregnancy. The same hormones have stimulated the growth of hyacinths, fuchsia, a meadow grass, the *reine marguerite,* white lupine, cooking onions, corn, pea embryos, hazel, and horse chestnuts.[8] Progesterone, another type of ovarian hormone, has inhibited the growth of lupine roots and hyacinth roots (Macht, 1946; Wasicky et al., 1933); relatively high doses of progesterone stimulated the growth of hyacinth roots (Cortesi et al., 1957). Estrogens failed to stimulate the growth of oat seedlings (Kögl et al., 1933b); there have been other negative reports (Thimann, 1948b). Several enterprising modern investigators have tested the ability of pregnancy and nonpregnancy urines to promote the germination of seeds. Manger (1933) found no difference in growth rates of barley and wheat. Hofmann (1934) reported that, over a period of a good many days, the sprouting of these cereals was less inhibited by pregnancy than by nonpregnancy urine. The Egyptian pregnancy test was repeated by Henriksen (1941) for fifty urines; he "obtained a 75 per cent correct positive and 85 per cent correct negative result," much better than would be expected on the basis of chance. A more recent trial of the ancient Egyptian method was conducted at a modern research center in Cairo. In these experiments, it was determined that nonpregnancy urines and about half the pregnancy urines arrested the germination of both barley and wheat. Growth occurred in the presence of the other pregnancy urines. The investigators "concluded that when growth occurs, the urine is presumably that of a pregnant woman, but the reverse is not necessarily true" (Ghalioungui et al., 1963). Thus the possibility of an empirical basis for the Egyptian test is by no means excluded.

7. Bonner and Galston (1952), Boysen Jensen (1936), Braungart and Arnett (1962), Kögl et al. (1933a), Rønnike (1960, 1961), Thimann (1948a), Wieland et al. (1954).
8. Burkhardt (1941), Chouard (1937), Macht (1946), Schoeller and Goebel (1931), Thimann (1948b), Wasicky et al. (1933), Zollikofer (1939a,b).

Another Egyptian pregnancy test depended on the failure of pregnancy urine to damage plants. In a relatively recent (third century A.D.) papyrus discovered at Thebes, it is directed that the woman should urinate on an (unspecified) plant in the evening. If next morning the plant is scorched, she will not become pregnant, but if the plant is undamaged, conception is possible (Griffith and Thompson, 1904). Dawson (1929) and Iversen (1939) regard this method as a variant of the pregnancy test already described. The latter authority points out that a very similar passage occurs in the writings of Avicenna; here the recommended plant is lettuce, and Iversen shrewdly relates the Egyptian hieroglyph for *scorched* to Avicenna's *exsiccaverit*. Sixteenth- and seventeenth-century writers recommended that the test be carried out with poplars, nettles, beans, barley, fenugreek, lettuce, or mallows.[9] Finally, *The Experienced Midwife* recommends as a fertility test that the man's and woman's urine each be sprinkled on a lettuce leaf; "that which dries away first is unfruitful" (Aristotle, 1793).

Other things than plants could be affected. Ryff and Guainerio recommended that a polished needle be placed overnight in a vessel of urine; next morning the needle will have reddish spots if the woman is pregnant; otherwise the needle will be black and smooth. The same test was mentioned by Jacob Rueff in his volume with the reassuring title (translated) *A Nice, Cheerful Little Book of Comfort Regarding the Hardships of Pregnancy and Birth of Mankind,* as well as elsewhere. Rueff and Roche both specify that the urine be placed in a bronze vessel. Culpeper in the next century describes what is obviously the same test, but with one important difference:

> Take a handsome green Nettle, and put it into the Urin of the Woman, cover it close, and let it remain in a whole night; if the Woman be with Child, it will be full of red spots on the morrow; if not, it will be blackish.

It would be interesting to know what misunderstanding caused the substitution of *nettle* for *needle*. Mrs. Jane Sharp's *The Midwives Book* (1671) repeated these directions (Brockbank, 1958). In his *Dreckapotheke* of 1714 Paulini attributed the method to Wecker (1587). The test also is described in *The Experienced Midwife* (Aristotle, 1793)

9. Beckherus (1660), Bourke (1891), Culpeper (1672), Guainerius (1500), Khunrath (1623), Rueff (1554), Ryff (1545). W. H. Ryff is not to be confused with Jacob Rueff. Ryff's *Frawen Rosengarten* was a plagiarism from Eucharius Rösslin (Rucker, 1946).

and, it is reported, in an old Icelandic scroll (Bartels, 1900). It was a practice in Hungary among the Magyars to stick a sewing needle into a picture of the Virgin and to leave it there for nine days. If the needle were then still clean, the woman had not conceived; if rusty, she was pregnant (Hovorka and Kronfeld, 1909). A Slavic variation was for the woman to urinate for three evenings in a row on the head of an ax, leaving it behind a door. Rust on the ax in the morning meant that a baby was on the way (Ploss et al., 1935).

Another urine test for pregnancy seemed to depend on spontaneous generation. A fragment in the Carlsberg papyrus (Iversen, 1939) gives part of the procedure, which is clearly the same as for a sterility test described in the eleventh century by that remarkable woman gynecologist, Trotula (1574).[10] The method required the usual two jars of bran, one to receive the urine of the husband and the other that of the wife. Sterility was indicated if worms were subsequently found in a jar. Albertus Magnus (1542), Guainerio (1500), and Ryff (1545) recommended the test. Rueff (1554, 1580) advised:

> A more certain experiment will be to bottle up the woman's urine in a glass for three days, at which time exactly it is strained through pure muslin, and if she has conceived, minute animalcules looking like lice will appear.

The same procedure is described by Roche (1586), by Culpeper (1653) who suggests a rationale ("if you find small living creatures in it, she is most assuredly conceived with Child; for the Urin which were before part of her own substance, will be generated as well as its Mistris"), by Paulini (1714), and by the pseudonymous author of *The Experienced Midwife* (Aristotle, 1793). Bartels says the method was used in Iceland (1900).

Quite a different test for pregnancy was to dose the patient with a potion and await her reaction. Vomiting was often a positive sign, as well it might have been; a queasy stomach is a common affliction during early pregnancy. The Egyptian hieroglyphs are again the earliest source of information. The Petrie papyri, according to Griffith (1898) date chiefly from the Middle Kingdom (about 2400 to 1580 B.C.) Prescription XXVII in this document is a fragment with crucial informa-

---

10. The existence of Trotula has been debated, but several authorities are now convinced that she was an actual person (Mason-Hohl, 1940). She is referred to in Chaucer's *The Wife of Bath's Prologue* (line 677; Skeat, 1924) and is sometime spoken of as "Dame Trot" (Garrison, 1929, p. 150).

tion missing; we only know that the woman must lie on ground which is wiped with the dregs of sweet beer and that an unknown procedure (not necessarily taking a potion) follows; if she then vomits, she is pregnant, the number of times she is sick indicates the number of children to be expected, and if she fails to react she is sterile. Prescription VII (also fragmentary) of the Carlsberg papyrus directs that the woman drink a mixture including dates, wine, and *sermet;* other ingredients were named in the missing section. Vomiting is a positive sign of pregnancy; flatulence, a negative indication. This test, Iversen (1939) points out, obviously is comparable with Prescription 193 of the Berlin papyrus, which specifies a potion of pounded watermelon and the milk of the mother of a boy. Prescription 194 directs that this mixture be introduced intravaginally; the same responses are to be looked for (Wreszinski, 1909). Earlier translations give the ingredients of the potion in Prescription 193 as the *herbe batatu de taureau* or the plant *boudodou-ka,* bruised with the milk of the mother of a boy (Brugsch, 1863; Chabas, 1862). Renouf (1873) thinks that the plant belongs to the cucumber family (watermelon?); Fasbender (1897) translates the hieroglyph as watermelon seeds.

It is most significant, as several commentators have emphasized (see above), that the Hippocratic writings contain a very similar test for fertility: "If you wish to know whether a woman will conceive, give her to drink in the morning on an empty stomach some butter and milk of a woman nursing a boy; if the woman has eructations, she will conceive; if not, not." Another Hippocratic test was to administer powdered red chalk and anise as a potion, to be followed by sleep; then pain around the navel was a sign of pregnancy (Littré, 1844). Jacob Rueff, two thousand years later (1580) believed that vomiting after drinking the juice of a thistle was a sure sign of conception. German folk medicine advocated a comparable method. In Bavaria, apple, pear, or grape wine was allowed to stand overnight in a bowl; if the woman drank it and then vomited, she was pregnant (Lammert, 1869). Arab women in Algeria were told to drink a red liquid made by boiling the crushed roots of madder (*Rubia tinctorum*). If her next urine was red, she was not considered to be pregnant, while urine of normal appearance proved that she was to be a mother (Hilton-Simpson, 1922).

Hippocrates' Aphorism 41 outlines another test. The woman eats no supper and drinks hydromel (water and honey) before going to sleep; she is pregnant if she is seized with abdominal pains. The test is said to have been suggested also by Avicenna; certainly it turned up again in the thirteenth century, when physicians recommended a mixture of melicratum (a kind of mead, perhaps identical with hydromel) and rain water (Gordonius, 1542; Johannes Anglicus, 1492). Guainerio believed the abdominal discomfort that could follow drinking the potion was due to compression of the viscera by the pregnant uterus (1500), an idea he may have obtained from Avicenna (Wolff, 1586). This method of diagnosing approaching motherhood was popular in the fifteenth century and later—"8 oz. of rain water to 4 oz. of honey. Boil until a third part is consumed." [11] Honey, curiously was one of the several substances believed in Austria to produce infertility if swallowed at the end of menstruation; other things taken by the credulous for the same purpose were tincture of cinnamon, English balsam, and purgatives of myrrh and aloes (Fossel, 1886).

When a twentieth-century gynecologist is dealing with a case of suspected infertility, he may introduce carbon dioxide gas into the uterine cervix through a cannula (Rubin or tubal insufflation test), meanwhile watching a manometer to see if a rise in gas pressure indicates that the carbon dioxide is unable to traverse the cavities of the uterus and Fallopian tubes and escape into the abdomen. At the same time he listens with his stethoscope for the sound of gas leaving the tubes. His purpose is to determine whether obstructions in the tubes are preventing the descent and fertilization of ova, thus causing sterility.

The Egyptians had reasoned also that obstruction of the uterus would make it impossible for a woman to have a child. Their simple and ingenious test seems to have been based on the erroneous idea that the cavity of the uterus somehow communicated with that of the digestive tract and ultimately with the mouth and nose. As early as the Twelfth Dynasty (about 2000 to 1800 B.C.), the fragmentary Prescription IV of the Carlsberg papyrus, as interpreted by Iversen (1939), directed that an onion bulb be allowed to remain all night in the vagina. If in the morning the woman can taste the onion, "she will give birth." The even more incomplete Prescription XXVIII of the Petrie papyri seems to be almost identical (Griffith, 1898). Iversen directs attention to the closely parallel Hippocratic prescription: peel the outer layers from a piece of garlic and apply it as a pessary; if in the

11. Savanarola (1560, 1561). See also Albertus Magnus (1580), Arnaldus (1494), Bonaciolus (1563), Candidus (1498), Culpeper (1676), Malgaigne (1840), Roche (1586), Rösslin (1513), Rueff (1554), Ryff (1545), Sudhoff (1916).

morning the woman tastes the garlic, she will conceive (Littré, 1844). Or the pessary may be of wool containing a little *netopon* (oil of bitter almonds). Or a strongly flavored substance may travel in the reverse direction: if she drinks anise pounded in water and then experiences itching in the region of the navel, she will conceive. Hippocrates further suggests that the lower part of the woman's body could be swathed in blankets and fumigated; "and if it appear that the scent passes through the body to the nostrils and mouth, know that of herself she is not unfruitful" (Adams, 1849). Priscian in the fourth century A.D. suggested a suppository of *galbanum,* an aromatic resin resembling asafetida; if the top of the woman's head then became warm, she could become pregnant (Priscianus et al., 1597). Although these methods were based on gross misunderstanding of human anatomy, they all seem to represent attempts to obtain the answer to a reasonable question—is the uterus open so that pregnancy can occur?

By the time John of Gaddesden described the suppository method, it was presented as a test not for fertility but for pregnancy. A regimen prescribed in the fifteenth century for "the illustrious Lady Margaretha, Markgräfin of Brandenburg," directed that a piece of garlic be used and that the lady then fast for a whole day. If the next morning she could taste the garlic, she would conceive (Sudhoff, 1916).

Bernard de Gordon reversed the Hippocratic interpretation. He described fumigation with an aromatic substance and stated that if the woman detected the odor she was not pregnant (Gordon, 1542).

Prescriptions for fumigation were turned up by Wilde (1849) in ancient Irish writings, particularly in a copy made in 1496 of a book by Fiongan MacTully, a hereditary physician of the province of Connaught. One procedure is "To burn the meal of Darnel (a grass) and frankincense on a red stone, and let the smoke pass through a funnel under her (a woman), and that will prepare her for conception." Wilde recognized that the prescription probably came from a classic author. Dioscorides (1598 ed.), a physician of the first century A.D., had, as Wilde points out, recommended fumigating with a mixture of darnel, "barley flour, myrhh, saffron or frankincense as an aid to conception." Other Irish mixtures to be used in fumigation to promote (not to test for) conception were steam from the oriental narcissus (?) boiled in wine or water, or smoke from this plant burned on a red stone. Clearly, as often happened with the passage of years, the Egyptian and Hippocratic idea had again been misunderstood, and fumigation was here being used therapeutically rather than diagnostically.

Guainerio precribed fumigation as a fertility test in 1500. He also suggested a kind of medicated pessary composed of honey and *Aristolochia* or birthwort, the pungent root of which was thought to facilitate childbirth. The pessary was introduced before sleeping; the woman was judged to be fertile if on awakening she had a sweet taste in her mouth. Or, said Guainerio, she might simply sleep over a piece of garlic; if she tasted garlic when she woke, she would be able to have a child. Rösslin (1540) suggested:

> the fume of some odoriferous perfume / as laudanum / stozar / calamyte/lignum aloes/muske/ambre and suche other/yf the odour and savour of suche thynges assende thorowe her body up unto her nose/ye shall understande/that sterilite commeth not of the womans parte / yf not: then is the defecte in her.

Ryff (1545), Rueff (1554), and Bonaciolus (1563) recommended fumigation; Savonarola (1560) mentioned fumigation and pessaries of garlic and birthwort:

> 1 drachm. Let it be bruised and mixed with honey and buried [i.e. inserted] with green moss continuously until morning. Then at noontide, if while fasting her saliva grows sweet she will conceive, and similarly if it is bitter, if she does not detect its savor, she will not be pregnant.

Aschheim (1930) says Albertus Magnus wrote that if milk is poured on urine and if the woman is pregnant, the milk floats on top.

One is glad to know that not all physicians accepted such tests. Several eighteenth-century experts decried them.[12] The potion test had been condemned earlier by a medicolegal expert as not only fallacious but dangerous (Zacchia, 1674). To differ with Hippocrates, Galen, and Avicenna took courage indeed, particularly in 1602, when Fortunatus Fidelis dared to speak out:

> Truly Hippocrates has recommended [uroscopy] for the diagnosis not of pregnancy but of fertility. Avicenna is accustomed to put garlic under [the patient] while the stomach is empty. Then if after sleep she smells it, it may be determined that the woman is

12. Culpeper (1706), Kräutermann (1730), Schurig (1731), Teichmeyer (1731).

free from the influence of the uterus. Indeed I by no means condemn these signs which are cited by the illustrious authors of medicine, for their authority is great. But yet if I were to be put on trial in regard to pregnant women, I would never attempt that kind of test, as [such tests] are full of danger and can injure both the women and the fetuses. For who does not know if when intestinal griping is induced in pregnant women, if aromatic incense is administered, or garlic is given as a pessary, whether these can induce both menstruation and abortion?

The early Irish volume referred to previously describes a quaint fertility test. If a woman could throw a pebble up onto the top stone of an ancient cromlegh (sepulchral monument) near Dunkalk, and the pebble did not fall off the smooth, convex surface, she could expect to have a child. The total number of times she would conceive would depend on the number of pebbles she could lodge on the top of the monument. The number of future children was also predicted on the basis of the number of knots or vascular enlargements in the umbilical cord (Wilde, 1849).

A Nigerian procedure was one of the few in which the woman did not participate. It was the medicine man who put meal and water into a calabash, washed his eyes with a drug, and observed the answer in the water (Tremearne, 1912). An old Icelandic test was for the woman who was in doubt to let two or three drops of blood from the right side of her body fall into a stream. If they sank, she was pregnant (Bartels, 1900). The same test was known to Peter Bayer (1561). In Lincolnshire, England, it was believed that a woman who sowed parsley seed would give birth (Rudkin, 1936). A small tablet of lime wood served the gypsies of the Danube area as a predictor. Burned into the wood were the figures of sun, moon, and stars, encircled by a snake. Wedged into a hole at the top was a hazelnut, around which were braided hairs from a donkey's tail. If the nut fell out, the owner of the tablet could expect to have a child (Ploss et al., 1935; Weissbart, 1905).

In a year when there were many mountain-ash berries or many hazelnuts in Germany, it was anticipated that there would be many children (Hansemann, 1914).

At least one pregnancy test was conducted in public. In a parish of Cumberland, England, it was the custom a hundred years ago for the wives of a neighborhood to be invited to tea on the day after a christening by the new mother. After the party, the husbands came to take their wives home. First, however, each departing female guest had to jump over a pail placed on the door sill. If she stumbled or put her foot into the pail, all her friends knew that she was in an "interesting way" (Ratcliffe, 1876).

Animals and birds, too, might foretell a pregnancy. In Hungary, it was a positive sign if a cat's coat was flat on the sides; in Bohemia, if a mole burrowed near the house; along the Danube, if a woman was licked by an ox or if a cicada lit on her. And both storks and owls had a message if seen or heard often near a home.[13]

A good many methods for the recognition of pregnancy and fertility involved certain physical signs. The obvious indications of pregnancy have of course been known since antiquity. Other signs, real or fancied, are both more subtle and less familiar. The Berlin papyrus suggested rubbing the woman's arms and shoulders with oil and next morning examining and palpating her arm muscles. "If the muscles of her arm thereupon contract in your hand, then you say: She has conceived." Other methods were to observe her superficial blood vessels or feel her pulse. The Petrie papyri gave a vague direction for examination of the chest muscles. As Dawson has pointed out, the authors of both the Berlin and the Petrie papyri regarded a greenish cast of the skin as a sign of pregnancy. A warm neck and a cold back were sure indications of conception.[14]

> When a woman is lying on her back in bed, if she extends both hands above her abdomen lateral to the umbilicus, observe carefully; if she is pregnant she will feel under her hands a movement as if of spiders, and a beating, especially if she is pregnant for only a short time. [Bayrus, 1561]

The Chinese are said to have diagnosed pregnancy on the basis of amenorrhea and a particular type of pulse (Diepgen, 1937; Gruner, 1930).

The great Albertus Magnus felt that a desire, now called *pica*,[15] for strange and unnatural foods was a sign that conception had occurred

13. Hansemann (1914), Ploss et al. (1935), Sébillot (1906), Temesváry (1900).
14. Brugsch (1863), Dawson (1929), Fasbender (1897), Griffith (1898), Lüring (1888), Renouf (1873).
15. *Pica* is the Latin word for magpie, a bird notorious for its habit of gathering up all kinds of unusual objects. Soranus gives a classical description of pica (Temkin, 1956, p. 49 ff).

(1580); certainly this symptom is seen sometimes in a pregnant woman. In Austria and Czechoslovakia, yawning disclosed an early conception; sneezing, its failure. Freckles or golden flecks on the skin were also considered reliable indications that a baby was on the way,[16] a curious idea when one thinks of how common freckling also is in children and men. Skin pigmentation is often altered in pregnancy (Greenhill, 1951), but the changes could scarcely be regarded as golden flecks. Aristotle described a test in which the woman's eye [lids] are rubbed with "red stone [red chalk?]"; if the substance penetrates, she is pregnant; if not, not" (Littré, 1844). It is interesting that there was a Czechoslovakian superstition that if a woman rubbed her eyelids until they were red, it was a sign of pregnancy (Hovorka and Kronfeld, 1909). Michael Scot (1665) said that a pregnant woman's eyes are more clear and that her saliva is more viscous.

There has been a good deal of speculation about another "eye test." The Berlin and Carlsberg medical papyri give almost identical instructions: examine the woman's eyes while she stands in the doorway. If one eye looks like that of an Asiatic and the other like that of a Negro, she is not pregnant, but if both have the same color, then the test is positive (Iversen, 1939; Wreszinski, 1909). Wreszinski suggests that the woman is made to stand in the doorway so that the light will be good without the sun shining in her eyes. Lüring (1888) implies in his translation that the examiner himself stands outside the house, i.e. with the light at his back. Since the eyes of the Egyptian, the Asiatic, and the Negro are dark anyway, the "difference" must have been rather subtle at best.

Classical physicians had another physical sign that does have a basis in reality; they knew that the neck swells during gestation. In suspected pregnancy, the diameter of the neck was measured daily. This procedure must have been common knowledge; Catullus refers to it.[17] The same idea appeared in the eighteenth-century French medical literature: "A girl is a virgin when a thread which has been stretched from the tip of the nose to the end of the sagittal suture, at the point where it joins the lambdoidal, can then encircle her neck." [18] Here, in-

16. Demič (1889), Engelmann (1884), Fossel (1886), Hovorka and Kronfeld (1909), Ploss et al. (1935).
17. *Carmina*, LXIV, 376–77 (Burton and Smithers, 1928). See also Garrison (1922), McKee (1886).
18. Pinaeus (1563). Guérin (1929) quotes the same passage from Deveaux' book on surgery (1743).

deed, a reputation might hang by a thread! Tait believes that Natalis Guillot was the first to discover that enlargement of the neck in pregnant women is due to thyroid hypertrophy; Guillot described the postmortem findings in two cases. Thyroid enlargement is now recognized as a common occurrence in pregnancy, puberty, menstruation, and the menopause.[19]

Although a few of the pregnancy and fertility tests seem to have had some empirical basis, it is apparent that a reliable procedure was not developed until the twentieth century. The failure of these methods must have been clear on the untold thousands of occasions when chance did not come to the rescue. That the tests survived, some of them for more than thirty-five centuries, is evidence of man's constant struggle to understand the phenomenon of his birth.

19. Marine (1935), McGavack (1951), Tait (1878).

4

The Prediction
of Sex

Undoubtedly man has from earliest times been gnawed by curiosity about the sex of his unborn child. Naturally, he devised "tests" to give him an answer. Until very recently, none of these very numerous procedures was reliable, but nevertheless they survived for centuries, probably because chance alone gives about fifty per cent accuracy in any large-scale trial in which the ratio is roughly one to one, as is the proportion of the sexes at birth.

An extension of an early Egyptian procedure, described in the previous chapter (Prescription 199, p. 37), is the oldest sex prediction method of which we have record. The Great Berlin Papyrus is believed to have been written in 1600–1400 B.C. but probably was copied from an earlier document dating from the Old Kingdom 4000–3000.[1] Many centuries later, Galen recommended the same test (Kühn, 1827), and about fourteen hundred years after Galen, Peter Bayer (Bayrus, 1561) still thought it was a good idea. So did Paulini, who included the procedure in his *Dreckapotheke,* along with the wry comment, "Women are always anxious to know whether they are pregnant or not—item, whether to hope for a boy or girl. If the doctor can give no reliable information, they have little respect for his skill" (1714).

Fifteenth- and sixteenth-century uroscopists looked for "louse-like" urinary granules; whitish particles indicated a male fetus; yellowish or reddish granules, a female.[2] More than a century later a French physician, Charles Guillemeau (1620), related:

> An honest young woman has assured me that she has tested this receipt, which is to take three fingers of morning urine and put it in a glass with as much red wine. Let this stand all day. If there

1. Erman (1887), Lüring (1888), Reinhard (1916, 1917), Wreszinski (1909).
2. Guainerius (1500), Johannes Anglicus (1492), Rueff (1554).

appears at the bottom a large cloud like bean soup, it is a sign that the woman is pregnant with a boy; if it appears in the middle, it is a sign of a girl; and if there appears at the bottom only the usual urinary sediment, it is a sign that the woman is not pregnant.

In 1933 a German pharmacologist repeated the Egyptian test on urine specimens from a hundred pregnant women. With twenty-three samples the germination rates of the two kinds of seed were the same. On the basis of differential growth rates of seeds in the remaining tests, nineteen diagnoses were wrong and fifty-eight were correct (Manger), a disappointing result. A more recent Egyptian study also found the ancient germination test to be unreliable in the prediction of sex (Ghalioungui et al., 1963).

Far back in history another idea developed which was to play a large part in later theories of sexuality. In the sixth century B.C. the Greek philosopher Parmenides said that male babies are formed in the right side of the mother's body and females in the left. This idea was to impress Hippocrates, as perhaps was also the belief of Empedocles (fifth century B.C.) that males, being warmer, are produced in the warmer part of the uterus (Burnet, 1930). The "Father of Medicine" (about 400 B.C.) described both tests and physical signs whereby fetal sex could be determined. He believed that boys develop on the right side of the uterus (i.e. on the warmer side of the body), and girls on the left. Therefore, he said, if the fetus were a boy, the right eye of the mother would be brighter and clearer and her right breast would be larger and of a particular shape. In addition, her complexion would usually be clear. If the unborn baby were of the opposite sex, the mother's left eye would be larger and brighter, the left breast larger, and she would probably have a freckled face.[3]

Pliny the Elder contended that a woman pregnant with a boy had a better color. If her baby was to be a girl, however, the woman moved with difficulty and her legs were swollen (Littré, 1850). Soranus, who lived in the second century, quoted (with some amplification) Hippocrates' physical signs, as well as others, but scorned them as unreliable and untrue in what is perhaps the earliest recorded skepticism regarding the prognosis of fetal sex (Lachs, 1903; Temkin, 1956). Galen (A.D. 131–201), however, whether or not aware of Soranus' rejection of the Hippocratic theory, seems to have fully accepted it (Kühn,

3. Fasbender (1897), Lachs (1903), Littré (1844).

1927). The authority of Hippocratic and Galenic tradition was enough to establish firmly the acceptance of the diagnostic signs by later generations of European physicians. It is of special interest that the Hippocratic criteria also appeared in an early Sanskrit text (Bhishagratna, 1907).

In the sixth century, Aetios of Amida, Court Physician to the Emperor of Byzantium, Justinian I, compiled most of the then current and recorded medical knowledge. He listed the Hippocratic signs with approval and added that a male fetus is more active and that its mother's blood vessels, particularly those under the tongue, are enlarged. Moschion (or Muscio), a sixth-century interpreter of Soranus, on the other hand, rejected the Hippocratic diagnostic signs as without value. Mahomet (570–632), it is said, endorsed an expanded list of the signs, as did Rhazes, Arabic medical writer of the ninth century, and Trotula.[4] The signs were recommended, along with other diagnostic criteria, in eleventh-century Anglo-Saxon manuscripts; in the thirteenth century by Albertus Magnus, Arnald of Villanova, Thomas of Brabant, Bernard de Gordon, and Michael Scot, astrologer in the court of Frederic II of Hohenstaufen; in the fourteenth century by Manoello, a Roman-born poet; and in the sixteenth, by many medical writers.[5] Hans Sachs, shoemaker, *Meistersinger,* and poet, outlined in verse "Sixteen Signs Whether a Woman is Pregnant with a Boy"; the attribution of the signs is to Rhazes, but the Hippocratic criteria are included (Göz, 1829). The embryologist Fabricius reported that the female colt develops on the left side of the mare, thus further endorsing the ancient Greek theory (Adelmann, 1942). Such is the awesome power of tradition.

There were a few unbelievers. In 1578 Joubert agreed with Hippocrates that a woman who will bear a son has a better color and a brighter eye, but pointed out, sensibly, that, as the human uterus has only one chamber and is located on the midline, the developing infant cannot lie either on the right or the left. Although Joubert's book was designed to condemn *Erreurs populaires au fait de la medicine et regime de santé,* he nevertheless speaks with approval of certain methods alleged to make possible the prediction of sex. Scipion Mercurio

4. Herrgott (1895), Mason-Hohl (1940), Ricci (1950), Rhazes, Trotula (1574), Witkowski (1887).
5. Albertus Magnus (1580), Arnaldus (1494), Bayrus (1561), Bonaciolus (1563), Candidus (1498), Cockayne (1864), Ferckel (1912), Gordonius (1542), Pinaeus (1563), Ploss et al. (1935), Rocheus (1586), Rösslin (1540), Rueff (1554), Scotus (1508, 1665).

sneered at uroscopy—"It is so false and lying, that it is more suited to charlatans than physicians, because the moon is more connected with crayfish than urine with pregnancy" (Bayon, 1939; Mercurio, 1621). The sex prediction tests were excluded from *The Female Physician* (1724) by its author, John Maubray, because "finding *they* tend only to *Curiosity,* and to no real *Advantage,* I cannot think it worth while to allow them any Place *Here."* But these men were exceptions. Ambroise Paré accepted the Hippocratic theory that each sex develops on its own side of the body, adding rather uncharitably, "The male infant is more excellent and perfect than the female, maintaining the authority and pre-eminence which God gave him, appointing him as chief and lord over the female" (Malgaigne, 1840). Culpeper's *A Directory for Midwives,* published in 1653, and Mrs. Jane Sharp's *The Midwives Book* (1671) also outlined the Hippocratic tests, as did such medical writers as la Brousse and the pseudonymous Aristotle in the following century.[6]

It is not surprising, then, that relatively recent studies of folklore likewise reveal the Hippocratic dicta, unrecognized but little changed, to have been widely accepted as popular methods for the prediction of sex in northern, central, and southern Europe, Japan, China, India, and Sumatra.[7] The Andaman Islanders who, after all, could scarcely have heard of Hippocrates, distinguished themselves by deciding that the movements of the male fetus are felt on the *left* side (Brown, 1922). A British physician made the same claim as late as 1891 (Ross), disagreeing with a colleague (Manchester, 1887), who reported that, during several years, every male child but one in whose delivery he participated had "been most prominent upon *right* side of mother while every female has been upon *left."*

Various extrapolations were made from the belief that males and females develop on opposite sides of the uterus. There was a Chinese superstition that if, after the seventh month, the right hand of the fetus pushed against the left side of the mother, it was a boy; a girl's left hand would be felt against the mother's right side (Matignon, 1895). Not explained was how the mother could recognize which hand she felt! Theodorus Priscianus, Byzantine physician of the fourth century,

6. Aristotle (1793), Chauvaud de Rochefort (1906), Culpeper (1653), La Brousse (1771), Sharp (1671).

7. Bartels (1900, 1907), Diepgen (1937), Eram (1860), Flügel (1863), Glück (1894), Herold (1953), Jacobs (1894), Karusis (1913), Lammert (1869), Matignon (1895), Moss and Cappanari (1960), Neuburger (1910), Ploss et al. (1935), Standlee (1959), Temesváry (1900), van Andel (1910).

suggested: "Let her [the pregnant woman] stand with her feet together, and if in walking she moves the right foot first she will have a male child; if the left, a female" (Wolff, 1586). The same test was later quoted by Constantine the African (1574) and others. Variants were to observe on which foot the woman stepped, or which hand she used to assist herself when she got out of bed or up from a sitting position; whether, when called by someone standing behind her, she turned right or left; which hand she used to pick up a key; whether she walked slowly or rapidly. These criteria appear both in early medical texts [8] and in recent compilations of folklore.[9]

If the mother's abdomen were larger and more rounded, or more prominent on the right, or if it were enlarged chiefly in its upper portion (European superstition) or lower portion (South Sea superstition), a boy would be born; if the reverse were observed, a girl. The mother was expected to be agile, comfortable, gay, and of less finicky appetite if the fetus was a male (but, according to East Indian belief, to be surly if it was a boy); if a girl was to be born, each maternal characteristic would be the opposite.[10] As recently as 1878 the placenta was said to lie on the left of the uterine fundus if the fetus was a girl and on the right if a boy; fifteen supporting cases are tabulated by the reporting physician, who nevertheless seems not quite convinced (Tuckey).

Hippocrates had stated that usually the female fetus begins to move in four months but the male, because he is stronger, in three (Littré, 1844). The great physician did not, however, suggest this alleged difference as a method of sex determination. Pliny the Elder contended that fetal movement begins on the fortieth day for the male and the ninetieth day for the female (Littré, 1850). The Talmud taught that the male fetus is completed in forty-one days, the female in eighty-one

8. Aristotle (1793), Bonser (1963), Culpeper (1653), Gordonius (1542), Göz (1829), Rocheus (1586), Rueff (1554), Scotus (1508, 1665).
9. Bächtold-Stäubli (1930), Diepgen (1937), Hastings (1919), Ploss et al. (1935), Moss and Cappanari (1960), Temesváry (1900), Trachtenberg (1939), Witkowski (1887), Ysambert (1903, 1905).
10. A very widespread group of beliefs. For earlier centuries, see Albertus Magnus (1580), Aristotle (1793), Arnaldus (1494), Bonaciolus (1563), Culpeper (1653), Gordonius (1542), Rhazes, Rocheus (1586), Rösslin (1540), Rueff (1554), Scotus (1665). For the nineteenth and twentieth centuries see Bartels (1900), Cockayne (1864), Diepgen (1937), Glück (1894), Göz (1829), Herold (1953), Hovorka and Kronfeld (1909), Jacobs (1894), Kaufmann (1906), Kéténedjian (1918), Lammert (1869), MacDonald (1883), Matignon (1895), Pickin (1909), Ploss et al. (1935), Riedel (1886a), Rorie (1904), Standlee (1959), Temesváry (1900), Trachtenberg (1939), Vincent (1915).

(Preuss, 1921), but did not specify that movements begin at these times. Medieval and Renaissance authorities were sure that the male baby begins to move earlier than the female,[11] and Russian (Demič, 1889) and Armenian (Kéténedjian, 1918) peasants have agreed. Daughters are more active in the uterus than sons, if Chinese tradition is correct (Vincent, 1915).

A reliable indication that the fetus is a male, according to Aetios of Amida, is to discover that the pulse is stronger and more rapid in the woman's right wrist than in her left; if the reverse is true, a girl is to be expected (Ricci, 1950). John of Gaddesden held the same idea (Johannes Anglicus, 1492). No doubt this superstition, which also existed in China, had much earlier origins. The sign is recorded in medical writings of the thirteenth and sixteenth centuries.[12] An exchange of courtly letters between two French physicians in 1771–72 set forth their arguments as to how, in the light of Chinese medical doctrine, the pulse should be palpated and interpreted in order to predict sex. The two doctors seem to have disagreed on whether a stronger pulse on the left indicated boy or girl.[13]

In the middle of the nineteenth century Frankenhäuser stirred new interest in this technique by claiming, in a paper delivered before the Obstetrical Society of Berlin, that a more rapid fetal pulse (an average of 144 or more a minute) during the last trimester of pregnancy foretold that a girl would be born, while a rate of 124 or less per minute signified a boy. Such a distinction, said he, permitted predictions *mit grosser Sicherheit*. Other physicians tried the method; some, but not all, were convinced. Modern opinion does not support Frankenhäuser's contention.[14]

In addition to the urine tests and the physical signs which have already been described, the credulous depended on other crude procedures, unscientific predecessors of modern, exact laboratory methods. In France and Hungary a delayed delivery was considered a sure indication that the tardy baby was a boy.[15] A sixteenth-century technique appears to be a modification of one of the Egyptian pregnancy tests.

11. Arnaldus (1494), Bonaciolus (1563), Gordonius (1542), Malgaigne (1840), Rueff (1554).
12. Diepgen (1937), Gordonius (1542), Göz (1829), Neuburger (1910), Rueff (1554).
13. Amoureux (1771, 1772), La Brousse (1771).
14. Chauvaud de Rochefort (1906), Cobb (1883), Cumming (1870), Eastman (1956), Eaton (1893), Frankenhäuser (1859), MacDonald (1883), Mattei (1876), Schenk (1879), Strong and Steele (1874), Wathen (1880).
15. Temesváry (1900), Ysambert (1903, 1905).

Pulverized birthwort and honey were mixed and applied on a pessary of wool. If the woman's saliva became sweet, she could expect a son; if bitter, a daughter.[16] Obviously this method, like many others, not only had no basis in fact but was highly subjective and hence was doubly fallacious. Paulini simply examined the saliva: if it was yellow or red and viscous, it indicated a male; if white and watery, a female (1714). A modern saliva test, although much more refined, appears also not always to be reliable (Ellin and MacDonald, 1956).

Galen suggested that parsley be placed on the woman's head without her knowledge; if thereafter she first spoke to a male, it meant that she would have a son. Priscian (fourth century) and Constantine the African (eleventh century) approved of this method, but Joubert listed the test among the *erreurs populaires*.[17]

Peter Bayer suggested that a grain of salt be bound on the woman's breast over night; "if the salt remains dry, she has conceived a male; if it is moist and liquefied, a female" (Bayrus, 1561). A modern German peasant might lay salt on the head of a sleeping woman; the first name she speaks after awakening will reveal the sex of her child (Bächtold-Stäubli, 1930).

It is a curious fact that none of the medical writers mentioned dreams as indicators of fetal sex. On the other hand, of course, dreams often had great significance for the credulous layman. In Russia, when a pregnant woman dreamed of a fountain or spring she expected a girl; of a knife or hatchet, a boy. A dream that the stone fell from a ring forecast the birth of a son but also his death. Dreams of the death of a pregnant woman, or of a knife or ax, were in Europe another indication that the unborn child was a male, while in India the same meaning was attached to dreams of lotus blossoms and mango trees.

To Maori natives, the dreams of the father are significant; human heads or skulls decorated with *kotuku* plumes mean a boy, while *huisa* feathers signify a girl.[18] In Southeast Asia, when the pregnant woman has dreamed of a number, she and her female friends sit up for as many successive nights as the number indicates, awaiting the cry of a bird or beast. If the cry is heard by all present, it indicates, dependent on the direction from which it comes, whether the child will be a boy (from the right) or girl (from the left). Should the sound be heard

16. Bonaciolus (1563), Johannes Anglicus (1492), Rueff (1554), Ryff (1545).
17. Constantinus (1539), Joubert (1578), Kühn (1827), Wolff (1586).
18. Bhishagratna (1907), Demič (1889), Diepgen (1937), Hovorka and Kronfeld (1909), Ploss et al. (1935).

from in front or behind, disaster threatens the baby. In this case the husband is quickly summoned to drive away the animal or bird. If thereafter the sound comes from the left or right, the child is safe.

In Albania the croaking of a raven or the nocturnal crowing of a rooster presaged the birth of a boy, while the cry of an owl told an Albanian or French mother that she would have a daughter. As Hovorka and Kronfeld suggest, girls could scarcely have been welcome; the owl's call was also an omen of impending death. On the other hand, in Dalmatia the owl's screech foretold a boy. African sorcerers informed the credulous that if a rooster looked at the door when he crowed, he was predicting the birth of a daughter. If he turned his back on the door, a son might be expected. Armenian women tore a hole in a cobweb. If the spider mended the hole quickly, a son was on the way, while a leisurely repair job meant a girl. And in medieval Italy the answer was sought from a lizard whose tail had been cut off. If the tail did not regenerate, there would be an abortion. If one new tail grew from the old stump, the woman would have a boy. A double new tail (which may occur) meant a girl.[19]

Medieval England had a charming test. The expectant mother was simply offered a lily and a rose. Selection of the lily foretold that her unborn child was a boy; the rose indicated a girl. If, as seems likely, she knew the significance of the flowers, then no one could blame her for so pleasantly expressing her preference for a son or daughter (Bonser, 1963; Cockayne, 1864).

Sometimes it could be learned from one child what the sex of the next would be by whether the baby first learned to say "Papa" or "Mamma," according to a superstition widespread in Europe. To cut the umbilical cord with a knife meant that the next child would be a boy, while use of a scissors bespoke a girl. Or the sex of the next child would be that of the first person encountered by the mother following her initial attendance at church after childbirth. If she met no one she would have no more children! A somewhat similar practice in Hungary was for the woman to put a distaff from the spinning room into her mouth and step into the street. The sex of the first person she saw would be that of her unborn child. In Saxony the woman thrust a wooden wand into the yarn on a weaver's bench, then sat on the bench

19. Amabille (1937), Bächtold-Stäubli (1930), Carič (1899), Delobson (1934), Hovorka and Kronfeld (1909), Kéténedjian (1918), Moss and Cappanari (1960), Sébillot (1906), Skeat and Blagden (1906).

and looked into the street to see from the first passerby whether she would have a boy or a girl.[20]

A famous test required a drop or two of milk (actually colostrum) from the pregnant woman. The drops were allowed to fall into water; if the milk then dissolved and dissipated, a daughter would be born, but if it floated on the surface, a son could be expected. Thus was the test prescribed by Aetios of Amida in the sixth century. Trotula said that either milk or blood from the right side of the body could be used, but gave the opposite interpretation from the signs. If the drop sank, the fetus was male; if it floated, female. A fourteenth-century English medical manuscript gave the same directions as Aetios of Amida. Johannes de Ketham's *Fasciculus medicinae*, now a rare incunabulum, included the method (the milk should fall into urine), as did authorities of the fifteenth, sixteenth, and seventeenth centuries. Disagreement continued as to the meaning of the sinking versus the floating drops. The procedure, also known to Jewish folklore, was in effect a crude test of specific gravity.[21]

A contemporary Italian test provides that if the drop of milk spreads quickly upon falling into a bowl of water, a daughter is indicated (Moss and Cappanari, 1960). In a variant described by Arnold of Villanova (1494) and by Michael Scot, the milk of the pregnant woman was simply examined: if thick, it signified a boy, but if watery, a girl. Or, says Scot, the liquid could be allowed to dry on a mirror or other smooth surface; if the resulting mass were compact, a male was indicated, but if the drop had spread, a girl (1508, 1665). A sixteenth-century authority advises

> But if ye be desyrous to know whether the conception be man or woman: then lette a droppe of her mylke or twayne be mylked on a smoothe glasse / or a bryght knyfe / other elles on the nayle of one of her fyngers / and yf the mylke flewe and spredde abrode upon it / by and by then is it a woman chylde: but yf the droppe of mylke contynue and stande styll uppon that / the whiche it is mylked on/then is it sygne of a man chylde. [Rösslin, 1540]

The instructions of another physician have a curious grace: "The precocious milk when drawn from the breast and cast on a glassy curve, if

20. Bächtold-Stäubli (1930), Chesnel (1856), Pachinger (1904), Ploss et al. (1935), Temesváry (1900), Ysambert (1903).
21. Aristotle (1793), Candidus (1498), Culpeper (1653), Ferckel (1913), Holthausen (1897), Paulini (1714), Ricci (1950), Rocheus (1586), Sharp (1671), Trotula (1574), Tuckey (1878).

exposed alone for an hour, is rounded into the likeness of the little glittering ball of a pearl" (Bonaciolus, 1563). The test evidently had a considerable vogue both in past centuries [22] and in more or less contemporary folklore.[23] Hippocrates himself had suggested that a dough be made with the milk and meal. The dough was then to be baked on a slow fire. If the cake burned, a boy could be expected; if it cracked open, a girl (Littré, 1844). Rhazes mentioned the same procedure (Witkowski, 1887).

A Transylvanian gypsy woman might break an egg into a bowl of water, then squirt water from her mouth into the bowl. Next morning she expected a daughter if egg and yolk were together but a son if they had separated (Ploss et al., 1935).

Divination was employed, as in the case of the medicine man who bathed his eyes with a magic drug and then saw the future in a calabash full of water, or who pinched a leaf cup of water and predicted a boy if the water squirted out (Hastings, 1919). Obviously the soothsayer could exercise his professional discretion and make a prediction that would please his client. It was a Slavic practice to study carefully the disembowelled carcass of the hog slaughtered for the Christmas feast. Soft fat meant a girl; lumpy fat, a boy. In this case, the interpretation was made by the men and women of the community (Ploss et al., 1935). Similarly, in the South Sea Islands the husband killed a young pig, removed the heart, and at the same time looked for an artery with a thickened wall. If he found it, he rejoiced in the prospect of a son (Riedel, 1886). An expectant Montenegrin mother threw into a fire a dried fish bladder. If it popped, a son was on the way; if it fizzled, a girl (Durham, 1909). A bit of bread served the same purpose in an Armenian superstition (Kéténedjian, 1918). At some Czech weddings the bride was given a blunt knife with which to cut a piece from a loaf. The piece she threw behind her. If it had more brown crust than white, she would have a son first; if the reverse, a daughter (Hovorka and Kronfeld, 1909).

A quaint tale came out of Denbighshire, Wales, more than a century ago. An old woman made a hole in the well-cleaned bone from a shoulder of mutton, knotted a string through the hole, and directed that the bone be hung over the back door when the household retired. The sex of the baby, she said, would be that of the first person to enter the door next morning.

22. Joubert (1578), Paulini (1714), Rocheus (1597), Rueff (1554).
23. Hastings (1919), Jacobs (1894), Karusis (1913), Pickin (1909), Rose (1905), Trachtenberg (1939), van Andel (1910), Wuttke (1900).

This rather vexed some of the servants, who wished for a boy, as two or three women came regularly each morning to the house, and a man was scarcely ever seen there; but to their delight the first comer on this occasion proved to be a man, and in a few weeks the old woman's reputation was established throughout the neighbourhood by the birth of a boy. [M.E.F., 1850]

An Armenian woman expecting a child sometimes heard an abrupt question: "Why are your hands dirty?" If she looked first at the backs of her hands, she would have a boy; if first at the palms, a girl (Kéténedjian, 1918).

In Brittany it was a custom to throw a boy's shirt and a girl's shirt into the miraculous fountain of St. Idunet or St. Gonval. If the girl's shirt floated longer, the child would be a girl, and vice versa. An Albanian practice was for the husband to slip over his thumb the esophageal sphincter of a hen, noting the diameter of the muscular ring. The latter was then soaked for half an hour in warm water. If it was unchanged, a girl would be born; if it had contracted, a boy. A startling Moroccan superstition involved dropping a louse on the pregnant woman's exposed abdomen. If the insect landed on its legs, the fetus was believed to be a male; if on its back, a female. A Hungarian woman would await a son if she discovered that she had burned a long hole in her dress or apron, while a round hole meant a daughter.[24]

The Malays cut betel nuts into pieces and threw them like dice to foretell the sex of the unborn child (Winstedt, 1925). In Central Europe, if a bit of the expectant mother's fingernail crackled when she dropped it on glowing coals, or if she found a needle (rather than a pin), she expected a girl. Or, early in pregnancy, she could dip a silver coin into holy water and place the coin on the big toe of her right foot. If the coin fell off to the right when she moved, a son was indicated, and vice versa (Temesvàry, 1900).

In China the wondering mother might resort to numerology. Calculations were based on her age and the phase of the moon when she became pregnant. With one formula, if the answer was an odd number she would have a son; if even, a daughter. If must be conceded that this method, at least, pays homage to the laws of chance. Sex prediction in Japan was also based on numerology. A South Indian superstition predicted that children born in the even-numbered years of the moth-

24. Avalon (1927), Bächtold-Stäubli (1930), Hovorka and Kronfeld (1909), Sébillot (1906), Temesváry (1900), Ysambert (1903, 1905).

er's life would be girls; boys, of course, could be expected in the odd-numbered years.[25]

An old French superstition has been noted recently in an Italian village. If a child is born when the moon is waxing, the mother's next child will be of the same sex. If the Lapps of long ago saw a star above the moon, they predicted a son, while a star below signified a daughter. In Touraine, to see a new moon within six days after a baby was born foretold that the next child would be of the same sex; if after more than six days, it would be the opposite sex. Or the crucial intervals might occur during the first and the last quarters of the moon.[26] Such beliefs perhaps derived from mythology, for Lucina, the goddess of light and of childbirth, was sometimes identified with the moon goddess Diana.

François Mauriceau, shrewd obstetrician of the seventeenth century, derides the superstition that a girl or a boy is conceived according to the waning or waxing moon.

> One can readily satisfy the curiosity and unrest of women who wish to know whether they are pregnant or not, but there are many who wish that one would . . . say whether it is boy or girl. This is absolutely impossible, although there is hardly a midwife who does not claim to divine it. Actually, it is better to guess it than to foretell it, because when [the prediction] materializes, it is assuredly more by chance than science or reason. . . . But one is sometimes so pressed and importuned to express an opinion, chiefly by women who have never had children, and also by their husbands, who are no less curious, that one is obliged to satisfy them on the matter as best one can, by consideration of some very uncertain signs.

After discussing and criticizing as fallacious a number of familiar tests, Mauriceau continues,

> If the midwife knows that one desires a boy, she will assure one that it is a boy, and that she would swear to it, and if it is a girl that one wants . . . she will say the same, and that she would wager it is a girl. If, by good luck, matters turn out according to her prognosis, she will not fail to say that she knew it very well, but when

25. Dennys (1876), Engelmann, Hastings (1919), Kershasp (1904), Matignon (1895).
26. Levret (1766), Moss and Cappanari (1960), Sue (1779), van Andel (1910), Wuttke (1900).

chance reverses her prediction, she gains a reputation for ignorance and presumptuousness.

The canny obstetrician adds (1675) that if *he* were the midwife he would do just the opposite, forecasting a boy if a girl were wanted, and vice versa:

> For if by chance the midwife predicted correctly, as could happen, [the parents] will say that she is a clever woman, and foretold correctly, and if it happens otherwise (as it will one time in two), the wife and her husband, having what they desire, will take little heed, as one always accepts cheerfully the good that comes unexpectedly.

A few other skeptics also raised their voices. The chief midwife of Augsburg, Barbara Widenmannin, for example, spoke her mind in 1735 in no uncertain fashion—"But whether a woman is pregnant with a little boy or little girl, no one knows but God alone." Nonetheless, there were always the credulous, and always a method that was supposed to be reliable.

In reviewing the numerous methods for sex prediction, one is struck, first of all, with that phenomenon noted so often in the history of biology and medicine, the overwhelming influence of Hippocrates. Even though he did not always receive the credit, his diagnostic methods continued to be used for more than two thousand years after his death. Another conspicuous feature of many old tests was their dependence on the body fluids—urine, blood, colostrum, saliva—of the expectant mother, tacit recognition of her influence on the unborn child. In the long centuries before the genetic regulation of sex was discovered, it was natural enough for many thoughtful persons to assume that fetal sex was controlled through the mother. Finally, it is clear that the criteria of many nonphysical tests of prenatal sex depended on objects identified, whether through sexual symbolism or otherwise, with the male and the female. In folklore, pins, knives, and axes were symbols of the man to be, while needles, fountains, and rings represented the little girl who would grow to become a woman.

The nineteenth century saw continuing attempts to find a reliable way to predict sex. More refined techniques based on scientific rationale and controlled laboratory tests were proposed, but still they had a disappointingly high margin of error.[27] Recently, however, one method has

27. See reviews by Blakely (1937) and Klotz (1947).

emerged which does seem to be dependable. This involves the application of the nuclear chromatin test to cellular debris of fetal origin in the amniotic fluid. The fluid, obtained by direct aspiration from the amniotic sac, is centrifuged, and the cells which have been desquamated from the fetus are stained and examined for the presence or absence of the nuclear chromatin mass which is predictive of female sex. The test can be applied as early as the thirteenth week of pregnancy and has proven highly reliable.[28] After at least four thousand years of effort, the goal has been achieved. Whether the predictions, now that they can be relied on, will make themselves widely useful remains, as a *Lancet* editorial (Anon., 1956) has pointed out, to be seen. At least one application has been found. Hemophilia, a hereditary disease of males, is transmitted to them through their mothers. In Denmark, permission for legal abortion may be granted when there is grave risk that the child will be afflicted with "severe and non-curable abnormality or physical disease." The nuclear chromatin test has been proposed for determination of the sex of fetuses whose mothers are believed to be capable of transmitting hemophilia (Riis and Fuchs, 1960). But hemophilia is not a common disease, and a scientific need for human prenatal sex prediction, as things now stand, would seem to be rare.

Thus the record of man's constant, driving curiosity to know the sex of the unborn child. Of course he need wait only a few weeks or months to have the indisputable answer. But in ancient Egypt as now, curiosity has little patience.

28. Anon. (1956), Dewhurst (1956), James (1956), Lin et al. (1960), Makowski et al. (1956), Sachs et al. (1956), Shettles (1956).

5

Chalcedony
and Childbirth

*It is also profitable to wear about them
gemmes and precious stones, as the
Saphire, Iacint, Corall, the precious
stone Corneola, Adamant, Thurchese.*[1]

The two chief lapidary authorities of the Middle
Ages, St. Isidore, Bishop of Seville in the seventh century, and
Marbode, Bishop of Rennes from 1067 to 1081, had much to say about
the curative and protective powers of gems and other stones.[2] The reasons for ascribing such virtues to these objects are not entirely clear, but
it is likely that the custom of wearing or holding an amulet during
pregnancy and childbirth is almost as ancient as the need for comfort
and reassurance.

The *aetites* or eagle stone was perhaps the best-known obstetrical
lapidary amulet.[3] Although not a gem, it was prized for a supposed
efficacy not only in preventing abortion and easing childbirth but also
in detecting thieves and poison and in treating epilepsy. The stone, in a
sense, is "pregnant," for it is hollow and contains a pebble, sand, or
other material, so that the aetites may rattle when it is shaken. The
stone has been known since the days of the Assyrians (Barb, 1950;
Thompson, 1936). Bromehead (1947) points out that there are at
least a hundred references to the aetites between Dioscorides' manuscript in the first century A.D. (Berendes, 1902) and Quincy's *Pharmacopoeia* in the eighteenth (1718). The "gem of parturient women,"

---

1. Rueff (1554).
2. Adams (1938), Evans and Serjeantson (1933), Fossey (1902).
3. I am particularly indebted to the authors of two excellent studies on the eagle
stone, Barb (1950) and Bromehead (1947). References in the literature to the *aetites*
are very numerous; not all will be mentioned here. Also see Aldrovandus (1648), Bausch
(1665), Evans (1922), Evans and Serjeantson (1933), Fernie (1907), Kaumann (1906),
Kunz (1915), Seligmann (1927), and Thorndike (1923, 1958) for reviews.

as Theophrastus (371–287 B.C.) called it, apparently was a related but different stone (King, 1865).

I confess to an early suspicion that the eagle stone was an imaginary object. However, one summer day in 1961 officials of the Department of Mineralogy at the Natural History Museum in London set my mind at rest when they kindly allowed me to examine a collection of eagle stones from Hungary, South Africa, Scotland, and China.[4] Most of them were of limonite, or brown hematite, and were up to three inches in diameter. When shaken, they rattled very satisfactorily!

The aetites was said to be found in the eagle's nest. Pliny gave authority to this idea; he states that the stones are of both sexes and that a male and a female are always found together in the nest (Littré, 1850). Lucan (A.D. 39–65), the Roman poet, perhaps with his tongue in his cheek, referred to eagle stones which explode noisily when heated by the female bird's body (1928 ed.). The male eagle (or vulture, in a variation of the legend) brought the aetites to his mate from India so that she could lay her eggs without discomfort. Thus Dioscorides, a Greek army surgeon who served under the Emperor Nero, a pseudo-Galenic manuscript, and other sources.[5] Bishop Isidore was convinced that the young eagles could not escape from the eggs unless the stone were present. He, like Pliny, believed that there were masculine and feminine varieties (Marbodeus, 1740). Bartholomew the Englishman discussed the stone at length (Bartholomeus, 1539). The aetites, added Conrad of Megenberg, also protected the eggs from the great bodily heat of the mother (Schulz, 1897). Icelandic legend told how to obtain a *Lausnarsteinn* or *Lösestein:* one finds an eagle's nest and binds the beaks of the young. When the father returns and sees their predicament, he at once flies off, coming back with several stones of different colors. He touches one after another to the bound beaks; the one that frees them is the *Lösestein.* Such objects are now believed to be the dried fruit of the plant *Mimosa scandens,* washed up on the coast of Iceland (Maurer, 1860.)

Pliny described four varieties of aetites, coming from Africa (a female stone), Arabia (a male), Cyprus, and Taphiusa. He also mentioned the *cyitis,* which contains an embryo stone, and the *gassinade,* which conceives, as does the *gaeanis* or *paeanitis* (Littré, 1850). His

4. Numbers 49140, 54277, 58168, 61219, 90322, and 191622 in the Department's collection.
5. Berendes (1902), Ruska (1896), Thorndike (1963), Vincentius (1624).

ideas were repeated, sometimes with embellishments, for at least 1,600 years.

Bromehead has summarized various descriptions of the appearance of the eagle stone, beginning with that of Bishop Isidore. In addition to the authorities he lists, Agricola, Thomas Bartholin, and Bayer also give careful accounts, based mostly on Pliny. Gesner distinguished among the *geodes,* containing earth, the *aetites,* enclosing sand or a stone, and the *enhydros,* containing water.[6] Adams (1938), a modern scholar, says that the aetites is formed by successive concretions of various soluble materials around a nucleus. If the mass solidifies and some of the layers are subsequently redissolved, the central portion may be freed. The geodes contains free minerals.

Barb (1950) makes the important point that the "great majority of eagle-stones are iron oxides, either limonite ('brown' haematite) or haematite proper ('red' haematite)," and that the latter, in the ancient mind, checks bleeding "not only of wounds, but of menses also; it therefore helps conception and is a protection against miscarriage." Both Dioscorides (Berendes, 1902) and Plutarch (1855 ed.) believed that the aetites was useful in preventing abortion and facilitating delivery. By the time of these writers the idea had developed that the eagle stone actually attracted or pulled on the unborn child. Dioscorides directed that the stone be bound to the woman's left arm to prevent loss of the fetus but that at term the stone be removed from the arm and fastened to the hip. Plutarch explained, "the midwives place [the eagle stone] on the lower abdomen of women who are giving birth with difficulty, and they at once deliver without pain." In the sixth century Aetios of Amida confirmed this (1543); when the aetites "is bound to the left arm it holds back the fetuses in slippery uteri. Truly at the time of birth it should be taken off the arm and tied to the thigh, and the pregnant woman will give birth without pain."

The obstetrical virtues of the eagle stone were extolled by that rather shadowy Latin grammarian of the third century, Julius Solinus:

> The Aetite is both yellow and round of proportion, contayning another stone within it, which maketh a noyse when it is styrred, albeit that the cunningest Jewellers say, it is not the little stone within it that maketh that tingling, but a spirite. This Aetite *Zoroaster* preferreth before all other stones, and attributeth very great vertue unto it. It is founde eyther in Egles nestes, or else on the

6. Agricola (1657), Bajerus (1561), Bartholinus (1684), Bromehead (1947), Evans and Serjeantson (1933), Gesner (1586), Isidorus (1493).

shoares of the Ocean: but most of all, in Persia. Beeing worne about a woman wyth chylde, it preserveth her from deliverance before her time. [Golding, 1587]

The two lapidary-clerics already mentioned, Bishops Isidore and Marbode, gave similar advice, as did Trotula of Salerno and Albertus Magnus.[7] Petrus Hispanus, a Portuguese physician who was probably also Pope John XXI in 1276–77, stated that the eagle stone can be found in the stomach or brain of that bird (1576). Further embellishment appears in a work on the lapidary art by Sir John Mandeville, pseudonym of a thirteenth-century author of travel books. He said that the *pierre de l'Aigle* can be white, pale, or various shades of red, and added that it should be worn on the left side of the body (del Sotto, 1862). Sixteenth-,[8] seventeenth-,[9] and eighteenth-century[10] writers, medical and nonmedical, supported the use of the eagle stone in obstetrics. Conrad Gesner also recommended application of the aetites to speed delivery in animals (1586), and Bausch and others suggested that it would cure sterility.[11]

Dr. Bargrave, Dean of Christchurch, Canterbury, wrote in the seventeenth century about an eagle stone bought from an Armenian in Rome.

> It is so useful that my wife can seldom keep it at home, and therefore she hath sewed the strings to the knitt purse in which the stone is, for the convenience of the tying it to the patient on occasion, and hath a box to put the purse and stone in. It were fitt that either the Dean's (Canterbury) or vice-dean's wife (if they be marryed men) should have this stone in their custody for the public good, as to neighbourhood; but still, that they have a great care into whose hand it be committed, and that the midwives have a care of it, so that it shall be the Cathedral's stone. [Jones, 1880]

On 4 February 1716 Sir Streynsham Master wrote to his daughter Anne, wife of the fourth Earl of Coventry:

7. Albertus Magnus (1569, 1637), Isidorus (1493), Marbodeus (1740), Mason-Hohl (1940).
8. Bonaciolus (1586), Castro (1662), Encelius (1557), Gesner (1586), Hervé (1906), Rueff (1637), Serapio (1552), Sylvius (1548), Varignana (1596), Vega (1576).
9. Ammannus (1675), Baccius (1643), Boot (1644), Chambers (1923), Culpeper (1654, 1700), Guarinonius (1610), Lovell (1661), Salmon (1678), Schwenckfelt (1600, 1603), Smoll (1610).
10. Aristotle (1782), Hartshorne (1909), Leonardus (1750), Männling (1713), Martius (1719), Mizaldus (1719).
11. Bauschius (1665), Evans and Serjeantson (1933), Leonardus (1750).

Yesterday I delivered to your grandmother Legh (of Lyme) an
eagle stone in an Indian silk bag, a paper sew'd upon it, No 21, and
in it a paper wrote upon—"Eagle stones good to prevent miscar-
ryages of women with child, to be worne about the neck and left
off two or three weeks before the reckoning be out." I had another
of them which was smooth, having been polished, which I believe
was that which you wrote to your grandmother about. It was lent
to Sir Francis Leycester's lady. [Raines, 1853]

In addition to these records left by laymen, there is testimony from
physicians in favor of the aetites. Candidus Decembrius, as Thorndike
(1934) has pointed out, said in 1498 that the stone had been used
effectively in childbirth on many occasions in the city of Milan:

My uncle Marcantius, a skilled physician, obtained such a stone in
the German Alps. I remember having seen it as a boy. He sought it
with the greatest diligence in the nests of eagles.

Another physician, Valleriola (1595), told of a patient from whom,
owing to carelessness, a large eagle stone was not removed promptly
after her delivery; after a few hours the uterus prolapsed, with a fatal
result. A noblewoman, one of Lemnius' (1658) patients,

wore this at her neck all the time she went with child, and was in
very good health, and when she was in labour forgot to take off
this jewel from her breast, she found presently a difficulty in her
labour, and that the child was slow to come forth. Wherefore taking off the Eagle-stone from her neck, and applying it to her thigh,
upon the inward part not far from the privities, she had an easy
and quick delivery. . . . By what vertue it doth this . . . I believe
it doth it by an attractive vertue, as the Loadstone draws Iron; Jet,
and Amber, draw straws and chaff.

A London physician, Richard Andrews, wrote to an expectant
mother, the Countess of Newcastle on 10 May 1633 that "I have also
sent you an eagle stone, which in the time of labour being tied about
the thigh will make the labour easier" (H.W.R., 1894). Mrs. Jane
Sharp, the famous English midwife, had, she said, "proved it to be
true, that this stone hanged about a woman's neck, and so as to touch
her skin, when she is with child, will preserve her safe from Abortion,
and will cause her to be safe delivered when the time comes" (Brock-

bank, 1958; Sharp, 1671). Popular enthusiasm continued, and the aetites appears in relatively recent times in the folklore of England, Italy, Russia, Spain, Palestine, Austria, the Faroe Islands, France, and Switzerland,[12] as well as in at least one book, Jean Paul's *Life of Quintus Fixlein* (Carlyle, 1858).

In addition to the notion that the aetites could protect against poison and was a useful remedy in epilepsy,[13] there was a well-established belief that the stone could detect thieves. Dioscorides had stated that a thief could not swallow bread in which (powdered) eagle stone had been mixed (Gunther, 1934). It remained for that shrewd and fascinating Neapolitan, Giovanni Battista della Porta (1910 ed.), to explain the empirical basis for the test:

> There is a stone called *aetites*. . . . Whoever crumbles it, and mixes it into unleavened bread, and offers the mixture to the thief, the latter is unable to swallow what he has chewed, wherefore the thief must decide whether to be choked or to be found out. . . .
> The real reason for this is that the [*aetites*] powder which is contained in it [the bread] is dry, so that the bread is made very dry, and pumice-like, and cannot be swallowed even with the greatest effort by him who has it in his throat. It happens that he who seeks to find the thief should say to the bystanders who are suspected to be thieves that he will perform a miracle, and he extols it vigorously, for then the throat of the man who has stolen is parched with terror and dismay, and thirst seizes him, until he in nowise can swallow the powdered bread, for it sticks to his throat, while if there is another without fear, he may swallow, although with difficulty.

Thus the unleavened bread, no doubt made even more dry by the inclusion of powdered stone, functioned as a kind of lie detector. The modern polygraph similarly depends on certain physiological responses which are controlled by the emotions and the nervous system.

A fourteenth-century list of the treasured relics at Durham Castle included, among other strange objects, "Item, a tooth of Saint Margaret, Queen of the Scots, one eagle stone, hair of Saint Mary Magdalene" (Baily, 1881; Smith, 1772). Some indication of the monetary value of

12. A. H. (1881), Canziani (1928), Hovorka and Kronfeld (1908), Krauss (1911), Pachinger (1906), Püschel (1963), Witkowski (1887), Zahler (1898).
13. Aetius (1543), Albertus Magnus (1569, 1637), Ammannus (1675), Anon. (1773), Barrett (1801), Berendes (1902), Boot (1644), Gunther (1934), Wright (1863).

the aetites has been recorded. In 1609 the stones sold for from one to twenty thalers (a German coin) (Bromehead, 1947; Boot, 1644). A news item in an English paper reports that on 21 September 1642, 150 soldiers under a Captain Scriven plundered Master Rowland Bartlet's house at Castle Morton, Worcestershire, of £600 worth of linen, jewels, plate, and other treasures. "Amongst other things valuable both for raritie and use took a Cock Eagle stone for which thirtie pieces had been offered by a physician but were refused" (Bartelot, 1923). Barb (1950) points out that Bausch's 1665 work on the aetites states that the current price of a single stone, with tax, in the Augsburg pharmacy was 16 to 24 *cruciatos;* in the Frankfurt pharmacy, 8 to 12 *albos;* at Freiburg-im-Breisgau, two *solidi.* A half ounce cost 12 *albi* at Mayence, 20 *albi* in Hesse, 7 *grossi* at Wittenberg, 10 *grossi* at Bremen. The *London Gazette* for 1–5 April 1686 carried the following advertisement:

> An Eagle stone tied up in a piece of black ribbon with two long black strings at the end of it, lost the 29th inst. between Lincoln's Inn fields and the New Exchange. Whoever brings it to Mrs. Ellis in the New Exchange in the Strand shall have a Guinea reward. [Bird, 1894]

One is glad to discover that at least a few physicians and scholars questioned the eagle stone superstitions. Gesner (1586) seems to have accepted all of them except for the idea that the aetites is to be found in the eagle's nest. Sir Thomas Browne expressed his doubts about the stone in 1646, but he was not sure enough to take action: "we shall not discourage common practice by our question" (Bromehead, 1947; Browne, 1646). Nehemiah Grew, cataloguer of the Museum of the Royal Society (1681), and Paul Ammann (1675) seem to have been skeptical. Robert Boyle, the British chemist and physicist, found it difficult to believe in the medical properties of jewels:

> For not only some of the Writers of Natural Magick, but men of note, who should be more cautious and sober, have delivered in their Writings many things concerning Gems, which are so unfit to be credited, and some of them perhaps so impossible to be true, that I hope the Believers of them will among the Votaries to Philosophy be as great rarities, as *Gems* themselves are among *Stones.*

Nevertheless, because eminent medical men had "inform'd me of very considerable effects of some *Gems,*" Boyle decided that he would not "indiscriminately reject all the Medicinal Virtues, that Tradition and the Writers about pretious Stones have ascribed to those Noble Minerals" (1672). There were more doubters in the eighteenth century.[14] Nevertheless, as late as 1887 (Witkowski) one prominent French mineralogist is said to have received almost daily requests for eagle stones from pharmacists in Paris and the provinces.

Surprisingly few references have been made to the use of diamonds as obstetrical amulets, perhaps because these jewels were too costly.[15] Rueff's famous sixteenth-century work on midwifery recommended the *adamant* or diamond (see the epigraph to this chapter) to prevent abortion. Among the home remedies listed in the same century by Charles Estienne, the French anatomist, and his colleague Jean Liébault, a physician, was the recommendation,

> [if] the pregnant woman usually delivers before term, it is good . . . for her always to wear a diamond on one of her fingers; for the diamond has the virtue of retaining the infant in the belly of the mother. [Hervé, 1906]

Rudius (1595) agreed. On the other hand, the diamond would hinder the birth process unless the gem were removed (Herlicius, 1628). The superstition persisted at least into the beginning of the eighteenth century (Culpeper, 1700; Männling, 1713).

Several stones now classed as silicon oxides were in favor from very early times. Bonner describes a red jasper amulet dating from the Graeco-Egyptian period. On the stone is carved what seems to be a representation of a parturient woman seated in a delivery chair (1950). Jasper amulets were also thought to increase lactation (Budge, 1930).

Dioscorides recommended tying jasper to the thigh of a woman in labor to hasten her delivery, as did Marbode.[16] Later in the twelfth century St. Hildegarde, German mystic and abbess of the convent of Bingen, wrote her "Subtilitates." It had a book on stones and a chapter on jasper:

14. Anon. (1773), Bajerus (1561), James (1743), Levret (1766), Pomet (1712), Quincy (1718).
15. Identification of some of the old names for stones with their modern equivalents has presented problems, partly because of erroneous classical ideas about the relationships of stones. I have depended largely on Dana's *System of Mineralogy* (1892).
16. Fühner (1902), Gunther (1934), Marbodeus (1740).

And when the woman bears her child, from that hour when she conceives it until she delivers, through all the days of her childbed, let her have a jasper in her hand, so that the evil spirits of the air can do so much the less harm to the child meanwhile, because the tongue of the ancient serpent extends itself to the sweat of the infant emerging from the mother's womb, and he lies in wait for both mother and infant at that time. [Hildegardis, 1855 ed; Thorndike, 1923]

Petrus Hispanus claimed that jasper would cast out the dead fetus. A Dutch manuscript of the Middle Ages and an Italian surgeon in 1500 endorsed the gem as an aid in childbirth. Leonardus recommended particularly the green variety with saffron-colored veins.[17] The stone continued to be suggested in the sixteenth [18] and seventeenth [19] centuries. Within the last seventy years, Greek and Bavarian women have worn amulets of jasper for protection from the spirits (Höfler, 1893; McKenzie, 1927).

Chalcedony (varieties were, and may still be, known as agate, carnelian, onyx, *lapis Sardius,* etc.) was one of the gems in a famous birth amulet kept in the abbey of St. Albans, England, since, according to one story, the days of King Aethelred II (968?–1016).[20] It was described as follows:

That devoted son of this church and brother of the chapter, Aethelred, father of the blessed Edward [the Confessor], King of the English . . . gave to God and the Church of St. Alban's this precious stone, which evidently consists of sardonyx, chalcedony, and onyx except for that which is concealed inside, the whole thing being popularly called Kaadman [cameo?]. . . . On the advice of those in charge of the goldsmiths' work, it is preserved and deposited in the treasury so that it may exercise its virtue at appropriate times. For it effectively confers protection on women in labor, and when sincerely invoked in the name of the Blessed Alban, first martyr of the English, it does not permit parturient women to undergo hazard of any kind. It is said, moreover, that if it is removed violently or fraudulently from the church just mentioned, the inner

17. Guainerius (1500), Leonardus (1750), Oefele (1899), Petrus Hispanus (1576).
18. Evans and Serjeantson (1933), Lonicerus (1560), Rueff (1554), Rueus (1566), Sylvius (1548).
19. Boot (1644), Castro (1662), Culpeper (1700), Herlicius (1628), Lovell (1661), Platerus (1666a,b), Salmon (1678).
20. Dugdale (1819), Evans (1922), Wright (1844). Miss Evans' excellent book has been a useful source of references for this chapter.

virtue of the stone will be lost. . . . Moreover, inscribed on the same stone is a rather blurred figure holding in its right hand a spear up which climbs a creeping serpent and in its left hand a boy holding his clothes to his shoulder as a kind of shield and extending his other hand against the image itself.

Evans points out that there is no indication the jewel was employed from the beginning as a birth amulet and that this practice may have been developed later. On the other hand, one can speculate that the spear entwined with a serpent and the figure of the boy may have been medical and obstetrical symbols.

Bartholomew the Englishman (1539) and Rueff (1554) mention corneola or chalcedony in childbirth. Lovell's formidable *Panmineralogicon* (1661) says that *"Corneol. Sardius* . . . applied preserveth the birth."￼ As recently as the first decade of the present century, carnelians and the white variety of chalcedony were valued by Russian, Bavarian, and Italian women as amulets against miscarriage and birth pains and for increased lactation.[21] *Sardius,* a black variety, would, said Rueus in his *De Gemmis* of 1566, "dispel fear, induce courage, rescue the pregnant woman from sorcery and evil charms." Massaria, Claudinus, and Renodaeus suggested the *lapis Sardonius* as an amulet against abortion.[22]

Flint has been worn or placed in the expectant mother's bed to ease labor, and rock crystal in ancient times was mixed with honey and taken internally to increase the flow of milk.[23]

Of the iron oxide minerals, hematite, limonite, and sapphire were valued as obstetrical amulets. *Blutstein* or hematite, if held in the hand, according to Austrian and Talmudic belief, would protect the parturient woman from uterine hemorrhage and miscarriage.[24] Limonite (brown hematite) found use as a primitive Italian pregnancy stone. The lovely sapphire was believed to help prevent abortion, but Mrs. Sharp said that this gem interfered with conception if worn.[25]

Most famous of the iron oxide minerals was the lodestone (loadstone, *lapis Ortites,* oritis, etc.), now known as magnetite.[26] The idea seems to have been that the attractive power of the lodestone, as

---

21. Kunz (1915), Pachinger (1906), Ploss et al. (1935).
22. Claudinus (1607), Massaria (1601), Renodaeus (1631).
23. Budge (1930), McKenzie (1927), Saintyves (1936).
24. Fossel (1885), Höfler (1893), Krauss (1911).
25. Hastings (1911), Hucherus (1610), Rueff (1554), Saintyves (1936), Sharp (1671).
26. The Latin *magnes* is sometimes translated as *magnet,* but it seems probable that reference was actually to the mineral magnetite, which possesses magnetic attraction.

demonstrated by its effect on iron, could serve either to hold the fetus within the body, thus preventing abortion, or to draw the infant forth, thus expediting delivery. Trotula advised the woman in labor to hold such a stone in her right hand (Mason-Hohl, 1940). Similar counsel was given by Petrus Hispanus and John of Gaddesden in the thirteenth century,[27] by Guainerio (1500) in the fifteenth, and by a long series of sixteenth-[28] and seventeenth-century[29] and even later authorities (Aristotle, 1782; Barrett, 1801). There was disagreement whether the amulet should be held in the right or the left hand. One expert said that the lodestone helped conception (Sharp, 1671); another, that it would *prevent* pregnancy (Damigeron, 1855). Hucherus included the *lapid. magnet.* in a prescription for a plaster to prevent abortion:

> Take of pure laudanum 2 drachms, of aromatic calamus, Armenian bole [a kind of clay], dragon's blood [a resin], sealed earth, lodestone, red coral, pomegranate rind each 1½ drachms, of acacia, cytinus [an astringent plant] each ½ drachm, of naval pitch and gum arabic each ½ ounce, of turpentine as much as suffices to make a plaster.

Malachite, a carbonate, had some reputation as a birth charm; it was tied onto the woman's abdomen.[30]

Of the silicate group, jade (nephrite, green jasper, etc.) was valued in Egyptian times and also was recommended by Dioscorides as a childbirth amulet. It was worn by Brazilian Indians to protect against illness, snakebite, and difficult labor. Jade, fastened to the shoulder of the parturient woman, is still an amulet in Bavaria, China, and India.[31]

Beryl, said Leonardus (1750), "is a Stone of an Olive Colour, or like Sea Water. . . . It helps pregnant Women in preventing abortive births, and other Incommodities to which they are liable."

The emerald (*smaragdus*), splendid member of the beryl family, was listed by Guainerio in 1500 as one of the gems recommended by still earlier authorities for use in difficult labor. Paracelsus prescribed it (Waite, 1894):

27. Evans (1922), Kunz (1915), Petrus Hispanus (1576).
28. Bayrus (1561), Capivaccius (1594), Leonardus (1750), Ronsseus (1594).
29. Culpeper (1700), Herlicius (1628), Massaria (1601), Nicols (1653).
30. Budge (1930), Seligmann (1927), Villiers (1927).
31. Budge (1930), Fühner (1902), Martius (1867), Seligmann (1927), Stemplinger (1925).

The Emerald strengthens women in labor, and is the sovereign arcanum for their ailments if prepared by distillation, [in the same way] as crystal

    ℞ Of the said Emerald prepared, ℈j [one scruple]

    Of the Liquor of Melissa, ℨj [one dram]

    Of Southernwood, ℨij [two drams]

    Mix. The dose is from three to six drops.

The more usual (and less expensive) method of using the emerald was to wear it on the neck, shoulder, arm, or abdomen during pregnancy and to lay it on the thigh during labor.[32] The gem was also supposed to prevent conception.

Several related stones are employed in the same way as the emerald— lapis lazuli ("if [hung] about the necks of women that are great, it preserveth from abortion, and is therefore to be removed at the time of delivery . . . it's used as an amulet to prevent swoonings in women that are great"; Lovell, 1661);[33] hyacinth (an ancient term possibly synonymous with sapphire; a variant name is jacinth),[34] meerschaum (Ruska, 1896; Varignana, 1596), turquoise (Rueff, 1554), and borax. Salmon's popular handbook of remedies (1703) includes the following recipe for women with difficult labor: "I gave them Borax, very finely poudered ℨj; [one dram] in Mugwort or Savin water ℥ iv. [four ounces] or in strong Wine, or some opening Decoction, or mixed with an Ounce of Syrup of Mugwort, by which they always found wonderful effects."

The galactite of ancient times, according to Webster, is unidentified. It may have been a calcium nitrate. In any case, it has since very early days been believed to promote the flow of milk, whether worn as an amulet or taken as a mixture with honey. Or it was pulverized in water, and the resulting milky liquid was drunk.[35] Some early authorities said they had seen "milk" flow from the galactite. Since calcium nitrate is soluble (it contributes to the whitish efflorescence that ap-

---

32. Bayrus (1561), Boot (1644), Claudinus (1607), Culpeper (1700), Fenton (1569), Herlicius (1628), Lovell (1661), Ruska (1896), Schroder (1669), Sharp (1671).

33. Boot (1644), Platerus (1666a), Rueus (1566).

34. Budge (1930), Hucherus (1610), Rueff (1554), Rueus (1566). Bishop Epiphanius of Salamis, d. A.D., 403 tells a wonderful tale in his *De gemmis* (Blake, 1934). Jacinths, he says, are found at the bottom of a deep, dark, and completely inaccessible gorge in Scythia. To obtain the gems, the flayed carcasses of slain lambs are flung into the abyss. Eagles that inhabit the neighboring crags smell the flesh, swoop down into the darkness, and carry up to their nests on the heights both the lambs and the jacinths which adhere to the bodies. Then the hunters take the precious stones from the nests.

35. Budge (1930), Littré (1850), Saintyves (1936), Seligmann (1910).

pears on new brick walls), it is quite possible that a galactite exposed to water would give off a whitish fluid. "If tyed to the Thigh with a wollen Thread, it facilitates the Birth of a pregnant Ewe," says an early translation of Leonardus (1750). Italian women regard a light-colored agate as a milk stone, associating *agate* with St. *Agatha,* the patron of lactation (Budge, 1930).

Jet, related to coal, was the *gagates* of the ancients. Evans and Serjeantson quote from the Sloane lapidary the recommendation that women in labor drink water in which jet has rested. Leonardus concurs.[36]

I was unable to identify four pregnancy stones. The *lapis Armenius* (Boot, 1644), *lapis Sidonius* (Hucherus, 1610), and *lapis Samius*[37] were believed to prevent abortion and make labor easier, while the *lapis Sarmenius* was thought to hinder birth (Laurembergius, 1627).

Lapidary and medical works often included nonmineral obstetrical amulets. One of the most interesting was coral. Hutchinson (1955) has recently discussed the significance of this material in various protective charms. Trotula (Mason-Hohl, 1940) recommended a piece of coral hung about the neck as a birth charm. Petrus Hispanus (1576) made the more usual suggestion for the time of delivery, that the amulet be tied to the leg. Several other authorities gave similar directions.[38]

Quite often, it seems, a prescription containing coral or pearl, or both, was prepared to be taken by mouth or applied as a liniment or plaster. *The Byrthe of Mankynde* (Rösslin, 1540) prescribed an electuary, or sweet paste, to be eaten if the placenta and membranes were not delivered promptly: "then muste ye minister such thinges to her the whych confort the head and the hart as be electuaries whiche are conficte [confected] with muske / amber / and the confectiō of precious stone / as Diamargariton [pearl] / and suche other." Walther Ryff (1571) urged a confection of pearls and other ingredients "to strengthen the fetus." For the same purpose, Bayer (1561) suggested that "The use of coral and pearl before a meal is useful," but did not explain how this expensive preparation was to be administered. Later prescriptions were more elaborate—and more costly. One contained

36. Emanuel (1867), Evans and Serjeantson (1933), Leonardus (1750). In Victorian days jet was much in favor for jewelry, particularly for mourning.
37. Leonardus (1750), Littré (1850), Lovell (1661), Platerus (1666a), Ronsseus (1594).
38. Aristotle (1782), Capivaccius (1594), Culpeper (1700), Guainerius (1500), Herlicius (1628), Piso (1580), Ronsseus (1594), Schwenkfelt (1600).

coral, deer's horn, ivory scrapings, sapphire fragments, hyacinth, and sealed earth (Hucherus, 1610). Trotula had suggested a drink made of powdered ivory (Mason-Hohl, 1940). Other prescriptions were even stronger:

> Preferable are cold pearls, mastic, finger bones, pulverized silk, powder of tainted poison hemlock, ivory scrapings, pearls, red coral; these having been dissolved with sugar in Sidonian [?] wine can be made into pills; [also preferable] are lozenges of ashes, sealed earth, confection of dogwood fruit, of roses, of service trees, with powdered pearls. [Claudinus, 1607]

Another prescription in the same book on the effects of drugs read:

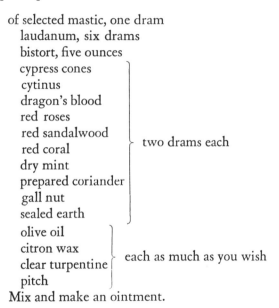

```
      of selected mastic, one dram
          laudanum, six drams
          bistort, five ounces
          cypress cones      ⎫
          cytinus            ⎪
          dragon's blood     ⎪
          red roses          ⎪
          red sandalwood     ⎬  two drams each
          red coral          ⎪
          dry mint           ⎪
          prepared coriander ⎪
          gall nut           ⎪
          sealed earth       ⎭
          olive oil          ⎫
          citron wax         ⎪
          clear turpentine   ⎬  each as much as you wish
          pitch              ⎭
      Mix and make an ointment.
```

Many of these ingredients are dry or astringent, or both. Since it was believed that abortions occur when the uterus is excessively moist, the fetus simply slipping out, it seems clear that prescriptions such as that above were expected to have a drying effect even if applied externally. Dr. Thomas Fuller (1719) recognized this fallacy.

> My Opinion is that Bole, Coral, Plaister of *Paris,* and the like, in Plaisters, do no Good, upon the Score of their being properly As-

tringents; for they touch nothing but the outward Part where they lie, and (having nothing of Volatile Steams) send no Medicinal *Effluvia* inward. But they make the Composition to be of a more Compact Body, and as 'twere better Mortar, to stick and cleave faster on.

Some prescriptions to aid childbirth, like the following from *The Expert Midwife* (Rueff, 1637), consisted largely of herbs:

> Take Cinamome halfe an ounce, the rindes of Cassia (or rather so much the more Cinamome instead of Cassia, because the Druggists often sell that which is not good), Saffron halfe a scruple, Savine, Betony, Maiden haire, Dittany, Fenegreke, Bay berries, Mints, of each one ounce, of the bone found in the heart of a Hart, Pearles prepared, of each halfe a scruple, mix them with sugar, and make a powder of them somewhat gross.

Nicholas Culpeper (1700) advised several preparations in obstetrical emergencies:

> If the water [amniotic fluid] break away too long before the Birth, such things as hasten Nature may be safely given or admitted, such are Dittany, Betony, Penny-royal, Juniper berries, red Coral, &c.

To prevent abortion,

> *Take Magistery of Coral a dram, Pearl prepared half a dram, Mastich half a dram, graines of Kermes* [39] *a dram, Manus Christi* [a cordial of sugar, rose water, and violet water] *with Pearl two drams, make a Powder.* If the Abortion be at hand, and the pains encrease, give this powder with a rear [rare, i.e. raw] Egg.

A somewhat similar preparation was advised by Jane Sharp (1671):

> Some remedies are specifical against miscarriage, and if the woman be in danger she may use them, and that in divers ways she may take them; as thus, take red Coral in powder two drams, shavings of ivory one dram and a half, Mastick half a dram, and one Nutmeg in powder, give half a dram in a rear egg. &c.

39. Quincy's *Pharmacopoeia* (1718), a most useful reference work, remarks that the juice of alkermes (or kermes) berries, "or the Confection made with it, is of great account amongst our Midwives, for assisting in Delivery." Much later it was discovered that the "berries" are actually the bodies of insects!

The pseudonymous Aristotle (1782) had a delightful recipe "to strengthen the womb and the child" during the first two months of pregnancy:

> Take conserve of burrage, bugloss, and red roses of each 2 ounces; of balm one ounce, citron-peel and Sheb's mirobolans candied, each an oz.; extract of wood aloes, a scruple; pearl prepared, half a dr. red coral, ivory, each a dr. precious stones each a scruple, candied nutmegs, 2 dr. and with syrup apples and quinces, make an electuary.[40]

Two other biological substances were sometimes mistakenly regarded as semiprecious stones and were recommended for use in midwifery. Bayer (1578) said that "The stone of ebony with which the goldsmiths clarify gold, if carried facilitates birth and protects the fetus without illness." Albertus Magnus (1569) about the same time, spoke of "the Suetinus stone, of a saffron color, which the Greeks call amber." It had several virtues including the easing of childbirth. Boot (1644) agreed, and suggested a dram of the material in wine, or six drops of magistry [precipitate] of amber in a potion or unguent. Dr. Thomas Fuller (1719) increased the dose. Oil of amber, he said, is:

> an extraordinary Medicine for Hysteric People, and is singularly to be noted for Women in Labour. . . . In this Case, I say, this useth to bring, as 'twere, Divine Help, beyond almost anything else, if 20 or 30 Drops be ministered in an appropriate Vehicle, and repeated at due Times.

An ancient amber childbirth amulet has been seen in County Clare, Ireland (Westropp, 1911). That such charms may have been in common use is suggested by a clerical injunction which has come down from the seventh century: "Let no woman have amber round her neck . . . or have recourse either to enchanters . . . or to engravers of amulets."[41]

40. Still other electuaries, ointments, etc. were recommended by Fontanus (1560), Fuller (1719), Massaria (1601), Platerus (1666a), Rhodionis (1526), Salmon (1703).
41. Wright has recently (1964) described a most interesting Graeco-Egyptian birth amulet found at a Roman-British excavation site in Hertfordshire, England. The small oval stone is red hematite (see Chap. V), carved in intaglio. The obverse shows a Greek palindrome and the *ouroboros,* the serpent with its tail in its mouth which represented eternity for the Egyptians. Other figures portrayed include Isis, a lioness, a representation of the uterus with ligaments and Fallopian tubes, and a key which symbolically unlocks the pregnant uterus at term. On the reverse are a scarab, another probable representation of a uterus, and in Greek the words *Orōriouth* (a protective spirit in gynecological disease) and, repeated three times, *Iaō* (Hebrew *Jahweh,* Jehovah).

6

Word Charms and
the SATOR Mystery

In addition to precious and semiprecious stones that
gave reassurance in pregnancy and childbirth, a popular protective device was the verbal charm. Sometimes this took the form of a Biblical
quotation. In Italy the Fifty-first Psalm was written on paper with pen
and ink as far as the words, "O Lord, open thou my lips." Then the
writing was rinsed off, and the water was swallowed by the parturient
woman. Or a paper bearing a passage from Scripture was hung round
her neck on a woollen thread. In Germany an invocation was written
on a wooden plate, after which the woman in labor drank the wine
with which the characters had been rinsed away (Ploss et al., 1935).
Eleventh-century Anglo-Saxon England knew a religious invocation
which was to be inscribed on new wax and bound under the mother's
right foot (Bonser, 1963).

The remarkable Arnold of Villanova (c. 1235–1311), a Spanish
physician who was also a lawyer, theologian, and philosopher, discusses obstetrical problems at some length and tells a quaint tale about
the method which "a certain old woman of Salerno" swore was nearly
always successful in inducing a delivery. The old woman used three
grains of pepper:

> With each grain she said one paternoster. When she should have
> said, "Deliver us from evil," she said instead, "Deliver this woman,
> O Mary, from this difficult labor." Then she gave [her] the three
> grains to swallow, one after another, with wine or water with the
> instruction that none of the three grains be touched with the teeth.

Then she said these words three times with three paternosters in her right ear: "Bizomie: lamion: lamium: azerai vachina Lord. Lord of sabaoth. Sky and earth are full of thy glory. Hosanna in the highest. Blessed art thou who comest in the name of the Lord. Hosanna in the highest." With these words in her ears, the woman delivered at once.

Arnold adds sternly, "I deprecate all this and believe that all the faithful should shun such diabolical practices and remedies" (Arnaldus, 1494).

Another prayer, read reverently to the woman in labor while a taper was held aloft, relates more directly to childbirth. It begins, "Ann bore Mary; Mary, Christ Our Savior; Elizabeth, John the Baptist. So may this woman, saved in the name of Our Lord Jesus Christ, bear the child who is in her womb, be it male or female. Come forth." (Lalung, 1939). A variation of the invocation, said to be popular during the Middle Ages, is written in the margin of an old book at the Monastery of Maria Laach, not far from Cologne. Translated, the notation reads:

> Excellent for a difficult birth. "Elizabeth bore him who went before, Holy Mary bore the Savior. Be thou male or female, come forth, the Savior calls thee. May all the holy saints intercede for this woman." Write this and tie it three fingers' [breadth] above the knee. If after this she shall not have given birth promptly, then write on another paper: "Lazarus, come forth, the Savior calls thee" and put it on the woman's chest. [Heim, 1893]

Another British manuscript, this from the second half of the fourteenth century, begins: "Boro berto briore † Vulnera quinque dei sint medicina mei! † Tahebal †† ghether ††† guthman ††††† Purld cramper †." Conventional Latin phrases follow. Here again apparent gibberish comprises a considerable part of the charm (Holthausen, 1897). The word *mei* was corrupted from *mea* to make this sentence into a rhyming couplet.

A manuscript dating from the fourteenth or fifteenth century and now in the British Museum states, "Here byginnes charmes for travayling of childe." What follows consists mostly of Latin invocations to the Virgin for help; an alliterative passage adds flavor and potency: "hora sedule sedebit, rubor rebus rarantibus natus nator saxo scik." The scribe adds,

Say this charme thrys [thrice] and scho [she] sall have childe sone if it be hir tyme.

Another. Say quicumque uult thris ["whoever wishes" thrice] over hir and scho sall have sone childe if it be hir tyme.[1]

Another. Christianum [?] age sursum erumpe et explica moras. Write this charme and bynd it to ye ryght kne wythin and als sone as scho es delyverd do it oway.

The idea here was to bind the charm to the right knee so that the infant would actually be drawn out of the mother's body. To avoid harm (uterine prolapse?), the charm was then to be removed promptly.

A fourth charm is an invocation to the Virgin (British Museum, Royal MS. 17 A. viii. fol. 47).

A quick and easy confinement was promised in another Latin document, a fifteenth-century manuscript found in an Austrian castle. The following words were to be written on a card, and the latter was then to be placed on the abdomen of the woman in labor.

From a man, a man; from a virgin, a virgin; the lion of the tribe of Judah conquers; Mary bore Christ; Elizabeth, although sterile, John the Baptist. I adjure thee, infant, by Father, Son, and Holy Ghost, whether male or female, that thou issue forth from thy mother's body. Be thou empty, be thou empty!

Again there is the warning that the card should be removed immediately after the delivery occurs (Zingerle, 1891).

It is scarcely necessary to add that, at least by the eighteenth century, and no doubt much earlier, the Church took a dim view indeed of all such charms—"vanity, illusion, and folly," to quote one distinguished authority (Thiers, 1777). Nevertheless, this superstitious practice continued. Even in the 1840s Irish women on the delivery bed still looked for help to lines inscribed on vellum which was then tied onto the abdomen. The charm, written in the shape of a square with crosses interspersed, enumerated various holy births and closed with the SATOR formula (Wilde, 1849), of which more later. Downright quackery was involved in the sale of a prayer to Irish immigrants as they left Queenstown. This charm was alleged to have been found in 803 in the tomb of Christ and to have been sent by the Pope to an emperor for his protection in battle.

1. *Quicumque vult* is the beginning of the Athanasian creed.

They who shall repeat it every day, or hear it repeated, or keep it about them, shall never die a sudden death, nor be drowned in water, nor shall poison have any effect upon them; and it being read over any woman in labour she will be delivered safely and be a glad mother.

Ulster midwives marked every outside house corner with a cross, then recited the following prayer before crossing the threshold:

> There are four corners to her bed,
> Four angels at her head:
> Matthew, Mark, Luke, and John;
> God bless the bed that she lies on.
> New moon, new moon, God bless me,
> God bless this house and family.
>
> (Black, 1883)

At the end of the nineteenth century in the Morvan district of France there were sorcerers who sought to accelerate childbirth by seating the woman in a chair, causing her to breathe the fumes from a decoction of mint and to swallow a dram of the herb dittany cooked in wine, meanwhile muttering in her ear, "Sus camp dur." The meaning of these words is not known (Bidault, 1899).

About a hundred years ago in Germany there was a vogue for the extraordinary *Himmelsbriefe*, or heavenly letters. Seyfarth has told their story in some detail (1913). The credulous were sure that the letters were actually written in heaven, then fell to earth and, of course, had extraordinary protective powers. These pathetic evidences of human gullibility were found on the bodies of many Saxon soldiers in the wars of 1866 and 1870–71. The simple peasants who bought the charms perhaps could not read; if they could, they may have wondered why German was always the official language of heaven. *Himmelsbriefe* were still found in Germany as recently as 1912. They were thought to give protection against all bodily injuries and diseases if carried on one's person. One promised: "He who has this letter in his hands and keeps it inviolate in his dwelling . . . on him shall I never inflict serious diseases or other major misfortunes." Another directs: "It is to be laid as a precaution in the bed of the spouse in labor and mother and then in the cradle of the newborn child."

In Dresden in 1908 a carpenter's wife was arrested on several charges including fraud. She had been selling "heavenly letters" for 20 to 30 pfennigs each, with the claim that they would protect the owner against disease and would expedite delivery if the expectant mother wore the letter on her breast. Related to these not-so-heavenly letters was another document of allegedly divine origin (printed in 1912!), the "Seven Holy Bars of Heaven." This also was supposed to lighten childbirth if placed on the chest or abdomen of a woman in labor.

A particular prayer book slipped under the pillow or laid on the head of a parturient woman was an accepted aid in the delivery room in nineteenth-century Germany (Ploss et al., 1935). A Syriac charm of the same period was prepared by writing "In the name of the Father and the Son, Lazarus, come forth" on a leaf. The latter was then to be swallowed by the suffering woman (Gollancz, 1912). Verses from the psalms were hung over the delivery bed or inscribed on the door or inside a circle of chalk on the floor. (Writing within a circle is an ancient rite of witchcraft.) The verses selected often were relevant to childbirth: "Get thee out," or "May he who harkened to thy mother, harken to thee also." Or the words were whispered in the woman's ear or written on a piece of cheese for her to swallow (Marcus, 1917).

But the most interesting charm for protection in childbirth and other hazards of this life was neither a Biblical verse nor a collection of gibberish. The sator formula, as it usually is called, is a word square. It has elements of an acrostic, a palindrome, and a magic square. An acrostic usually is formed by selecting a series of words whose initial letters themselves form one or more words; *news,* for example, has quite incorrectly been supposed to have derived from *n*orth, *e*ast, *w*est, *s*outh.

A palindrome (from a Greek word meaning running back again) is a succession of letters that form the same word or words whether read from left to right or from right to left. Palindromes have amused people for centuries. Here are two in Latin:

Roma tibi subito motibus ibit amor.
Signa te, signa, temere me tangis et angis.[2]

The first man in the Garden of Eden is alleged to have introduced himself to his mate with simple dignity: "Madam, I'm Adam." Not to be outdone, and clearly intent on having the last palindrome, she an-

2. From Kircher's *Arithmologia* (1665). Haverfield (1899) has described other and more elaborate Latin palindromes.

swered, "Eve." She could have added, "Name no one man." To an (English-speaking!) Napoleon Bonaparte is ascribed the sad reflection, "Able was I ere I saw Elba."

A magic square is one in which the numbers in a square are so selected and arranged that each line, whether vertical, horizontal, or diagonal, gives the same total. Athanasius Kircher (1602–80), the remarkable Jesuit physician, mathematician, physicist, Egyptologist, and musician, and perhaps the first man to search with a microscope for the causes of disease, discusses several of the squares (1665). Some are elaborate. One, "the seal of Saturn," looks like this:

$$4 \quad 9 \quad 2$$
$$3 \quad 5 \quad 7$$
$$8 \quad 1 \quad 6$$

Closely related are the word squares, which yield the same words whether read from top to bottom or from left to right. An early variant is "Abracadabra." Now only a figure of speech, it once was repeated in a magic triangle:

$$A \ B \ R \ A \ C \ A \ D \ A \ B \ R \ A$$
$$B \ R \ A \ C \ A \ D \ A \ B \ R$$
$$R \ A \ C \ A \ D \ A \ B$$
$$A \ C \ A \ D \ A$$
$$C \ A \ D$$
$$A$$

which was worn as a protective amulet. The "magic" lay in the fact that the same word could be obtained by following many routes through the triangle. Word squares that can be read in all *four* directions—up, down, left to right, right to left—seem to be rather rare. An example is

$$G \ R \ A \ S$$
$$R \ O \ M \ A$$
$$A \ M \ O \ R$$
$$S \ A \ R \ G$$

composed of two Latin and two German words (Haverfield, 1899). The great prototype of all such squares is the extraordinary SATOR formula:

S A T O R

A R E P O

T E N E T

O P E R A

R O T A S

A great deal has been written about this figure, in which five different words each appear four times as the rows are read from top to bottom, from bottom to top, from left to right, and from right to left. Much of the following account is derived from the outstanding studies of Guillaume de Jerphanion (1938).

In 1868 a fragment of painted plaster turned up in an excavation in the ancient British town of Cirencester, Gloucestershire. The plaster, from a wall, was carefully removed in the presence of the director of the local museum. On the fragment was the SATOR square, which had been scratched into the wall before it was painted. What made the find really exciting was that the letters were clearly Roman and could there-fore be presumed to date from the Roman occupation of Cirencester in the third century A.D. (Haverfield, 1899). At Dura, on the Euphrates River, in 1931–32 and again in 1932–33, extensive excavations of Roman ruins were carried out by a Yale University team under the direction of Professor Rostovtseff. One of the buildings in this "Pompeii of the des-ert" had served as an office for the *actuarii,* or clerks, of the auxiliary cohorts in the garrison then occupying the base. On the office wall, daubed in red ocher, was the square, in this case with ROTAS at the top and SATOR at the bottom. Again the letters were Roman, and again they had been written in the third century (Carcopino, 1953; Jerphanion, 1938).

The SATOR square had been found in other places too, in France, for example, on the pendant of a Bible dating from 822 in the Abbey of St. Germain-des-Près, in Egypt on a potsherd and on Coptic papyri, on a sixteenth-century Austrian coin, and in a book on amulets published in Frankfurt and Leipzig in 1692. The square was in the pavements or walls of churches—in Cappadocia and in Pieve Tersagni, near Cre-mona, Italy, and in the chapel of Saint Eustath at Gueuérémé. It was to be seen in the cathedral at Siena and in the Hamerslebenkirche near

Halberstadt. It was on a board in the chancel of Great Gidding Church in Huntingdonshire, over the entrance door of the twelfth-century chapel of St. Laurent, near Rochemaure (or Roquemaure), not far from Avignon, and in the parlor of the convent of Santa Maria-Magdalena at Verona. The square was found in châteaus at Chinon, Loches, and Jarnac, in the Hall of Justice at Valbonnais, and in a fifteenth-century house believed to belong to Agnès Sorel, favorite of Charles VII of France. And it was carved on a lead plate nailed to the cellar door of the oldest house in the little German town of Posneck.[3]

The SATOR formula was carried to many lands and appeared in Latin, German, Greek, Coptic, and Hebrew characters. Quite often it was copied or transliterated incorrectly. The earliest amulet on which it appeared is of bronze. Found in Asia Minor, this charm dates from the fourth or fifth century A.D. (Seligmann, 1914). The square was inscribed on buildings primarily to protect them against fire. To put out a fire it was a German practice to write the charm on a wooden or pewter plate, perhaps with crosses marked above, below, and on each side, and then to throw the plate into the flames. In a more elaborate ritual, the plate was carried three times around the fire, sometimes with the plate concealed under the bearer's coat, and was then hurled into the blaze. The directions emphasized the importance of running away as fast as possible. If one wished to prepare in advance for a disaster, the formula was written on paper and baked in a loaf of bread. Then in time of need the loaf was carried three times around the fire before being tossed into the flames.[4]

To judge from the variety of protective charms available, the bite of a mad dog was a much-feared hazard in earlier years. Here again the power of the SATOR formula was respected. Its use is recommended in *Libellus variarum medicinarum* (*Little Book of Various Remedies*), dating from the fifteenth century. The formula could be worn on the person or hung on a wall or tree. The charm was thought to operate therapeutically as well as prophylactically; if someone had been bitten, the formula could be baked into a cake or written with butter on a piece of bread and fed to the victim.[5] Jerome Cardan gave explicit directions in 1558:

3. Bouisson (1960), Carcopino (1953), Hirschfeld (1888), Jerphanion (1938), Köhler (1881), MacMichael (1905), Marqués-Rivière (1950), Reichelt (1692), Seligmann (1914), Villiers (1927).

4. Jerphanion (1938), Köhler (1881), Schwarz (1881), Seligmann (1910, 1914).

5. Frommann (1575), Hovorka (1915), Hovorka and Kronfeld (1908), Seligmann (1914).

When a person is bitten by a rabid dog, for three days he takes a crust of bread in such a way that, holding it transfixed on his thumb, you see the inscription [of the SATOR square] from the side; and five times while fasting he says the words individually in alternation with the Lord's Prayer, for the five wounds of Christ which He received while dying but not for the five nails,[6] as they say, and thus he is preserved safe from extreme peril.

Cardan adds cautiously, "So the matter is carried out, but the reason [for the supposed cure] is quite uncertain." Frommann (1575) quoted this procedure in his *Treatise on Enchantment* a few years later. The treatment remained popular, for the SATOR cure for dogbite was included in a nineteenth-century book of charms. This little volume, in fourteen manuscript pages, was owned by a German farmer. Tucked among its leaves was a piece of paper with the SATOR square written on it twelve times. The paper was already partly cut into pieces so that a square could be quickly torn off. The book directed that the square then be laid between pieces of buttered bread while one side of a post was marked with three crosses and the other with a star (Schwarz, 1881). In Brazil the formula was written on slips of paper and these were rolled into a ball to protect man and beast from snakebite (Hovorka, 1915; Köhler, 1881). SATOR was a charm too against wounds and burns, headache, cramps, fevers, and toothache as well as against evil-wishers, ghosts, and witchraft. The magic square was given to animals as well as man.[7]

SATOR was an important charm in pregnancy and childbirth. A protective medallion, one of thirty inscribed on a piece of vellum in thirteenth-century text, was said to prevent death in childbirth if the medallion was worn during pregnancy. The charm bore the words "Agios † Sator † Helyas † Hemanuel" and a figure of St. Margaret (Aymar, 1926).[8] Sometimes a book containing an account of the saint's life was placed on the chest of the parturient woman:

6. Cardan says *clauibus*, keys, but the context suggests that he meant *clauis*, nails.
7. Courtney (1887), Hovorka (1915), Hovorka and Kronfeld (1908), Jerphanion (1938), Köhler (1881), Seligmann (1914), St. Swithin (1905).
8. "Holy; Sator; Elias; Emmanuel." It seems strange that St. Margaret, patron of pregnant women, was a virgin. According to the story, she was driven from her home in Antioch in the third century by her father, a priest of Jupiter, because she was a Christian. Tortured and sentenced to death for her faith, she prayed for mercy for all those women who would invoke her aid in childbirth. The legend tells us that the earth trembled and even the executioner fell. In a heavenly vision she was assured that her prayer was granted (Albarel, 1924).

> Tenez: mettez sur votre pis
> La vie qui cy est escrite:
> Elle est de saincte Marguerite
> Si serés tantost delivrée.
> (Albarel, 1924)

The piece of vellum mentioned above was one of several found in a small bag owned by the Aurillac family in France and used many times as an amulet in childbirth. Another sheet in the *sachet* appeared, on the basis of the writing it bore, to date from the late thirteenth or early fourteenth century. One side carries many Latin invocations, written in thirty-four of the thirty-six squares into which the vellum is divided. A certain square says, in part: "Etz si pregnans M[ulier] super se portaveritz non morientur in partu †." [9] On the other side of the sheet are twelve magic circles for protection against specific hazards. One circle, inscribed to indicate that if it is shown to a woman in childbirth she will deliver,[10] contains the SATOR formula (Aymar, 1926).

The formula was written on the four sides of an amulet dating from 1259. The sheet of paper also carries in Latin verses four and five of Psalm 1. The directions state: "Write these letters surrounded with these words and tie them on the right hip of the woman and forthwith she will deliver" (Jerphanion, 1938).

A more formidable charm dates from 1475. "For woman that travelyth of chylde, bynd thys writ to her thye [thigh]." The charm itself, mostly in Latin, is an invocation. In translation it reads:

> In the name of the Father † and the Son † and the Holy Spirit †
> Amen. † By God's grace may the Holy Cross and passion of
> Christ be the means of my healing. † [11] May the five wounds of
> the Lord be the means of my healing. † Holy Mary bore Christ. †
> Holy Ann bore Mary. † Holy Elizabeth bore John. † Holy Cecilia
> bore Remy. † Arepo tenet opera rotas. † [12] Christ conquers. †
> Christ reigns. † Christ said, Lazarus, come forth. † Christ rules.
> † Christ calls thee. † The world delights in thee. † The covenant

9. And if the pregnant woman will carry [this] on her person, she will not die in childbirth."

10. *Hanc figuram mostra mulierem in partu et peperit.* Jerphanion (1938) points out that this corrupt Latin should read, *Hanc figuram monstra mulieri in partu et pariet.*

11. Again the Latin is slightly corrupted to make a rhyming triplet: *Per virtutem Domini sint medicina mei pia crux et passio Christi.*

12. Note the omission of *Sator*.

longs for thee. † The Lord of vengeance is God. † Lord of battles, God, free thy servant N. †[13] The right [hand] of God established goodness. † a. g. l. a. †[14] Alpha † and Omega. † Ann bore Mary; † Elizabeth, he who went before; † Mary, Our Lord Jesus Christ, without pain and sorrow. Oh infant, whether alive or dead, come forth. † Christ calls thee to the light. † Agyos. † Agyos †[15] Christ conquers. † Christ rules. † Christ reigns. † Holy † Holy † Holy † Lord God. † Christ who art, who wert, † and who will be. † Amen. bhurnon † blictaono †[16] Christ the Nazarene † King of the Jews, Son of God † have mercy on me. † Amen. [Anon., 1899]

The religious elements of this prayer are very similar to those in an Anglo-Saxon invocation of the eleventh century (Bonser, 1963).

The five lines of the SATOR square correspond to five Latin words: *sator* means "a sower," as of seed; *arepo* seems related to *arrepo*, "I creep to"; *tenet* means "he holds"; *opera* can be translated as "works"; *rotas*, as "wheels." Many scholars, of course, have tried to find a sentence in the square. Jerphanion (1938) says that the earliest translation is in a fourteenth-century Greek manuscript: "The sower is at the plow; the labor occupies the wheels." Another attempt was: "The sower halts the wheels with difficulty" (Villiers, 1927). A British correspondent in *Notes and Queries* suggested that *repum* meant "thread" in the fourteenth century, that *a repo* is two words, and that the whole could be translated: "Creative Power holds the wheels by a thread" (R.W., 1905). Further ingenuity gave rise to the suggestion that the twenty-five letters of the square could be rearranged to read: *Pater, oro te, pereat Satan roso* (Franco, 1881). This might be translated, "Father, I pray Thee, let Satan vanish by being eaten away." There was an Ethiopian belief that the five words of the square named the five wounds of Christ (Erman, 1881) or the five nails of the Cross—four nails for the hands and feet and one which attached the inscription. A Cappodocian notion was that the words were the names of the shepherds who visited the nativity (Jerphanion, 1938; Marqués-Rivière,

13. *N* for *nomen*, the name of the woman in labor.
14. AGLA is an acrostic from the Hebrew words *attāh ghibbor lĕ'ōlam ădhōnāy*, "Thou art mighty forever, O Lord." It often appeared in charms.
15. Greek: "Holy. Holy."
16. I have not found a meaning for *bhurnon* and *blictaono*. Possibly they are jargon; it has also been suggested that they have Rosicrucian significance (Whitmore, 1899).

1950). There were still other ideas. Certainly all these translations are labored and unconvincing. The great Jesuit authority, Athanasius Kircher, stated in his *Arithmologia* that the words of the square have no meaning at all (Kircherus, 1665; Zatzmann, 1925).

Then, forty years ago, there was a new and brilliant explanation, which, as Jerphanion says, seems of all the most probable. In 1926 Felix Grosser of Chemnitz, in Germany, showed that twenty-one of the twenty-five letters of the SATOR square can be arranged as follows:

```
                    P
                    A
                    T
                    E
                    R
  P   A   T   E   R   N   O   S   T   E   R
                    O
                    S
                    T
                    E
                    R
```

Thus the first two words of the Lord's Prayer form a cross. Two A's and two O's are left; they can be added at the extremities of the two members. If *A* and *O* are considered to represent Alpha and Omega, "the beginning and the end," still another element of Christian symbolism is added.[17] The SATOR square, then, would conceal within it three of the most fundamental elements of Christian belief—the cross, the Lord's Prayer, and representations of the infinite nature of God (Grosser, 1926).

Now it is well known, particularly from the *graffiti,* or wall markings, in the catacombs that the early Christians, persecuted at every turn and constantly in peril for their belief, employed several symbols with hidden meanings understood only by members of the group. (It

---

17. "I am Alpha and Omega, the beginning and the end, the first and the last" (Rev. 22:13). The equivalence in the SATOR square of A and O with A and Ω is discussed by Guarducci (1958).

is interesting to speculate, incidentally, that the Roman soldiers who drew the SATOR squares at Dura and at Cirencester were themselves Christians.) Perhaps the best known of these signs was ⟨✗ , the fish. This could be drawn quickly in the dust, and as quickly be erased. The Greek word for fish is *ichthys*, ιχθυς. This is also an acrostic for the initials of Greek words which may be translated, "Jesus Christ, the Son of God, Saviour." Like SATOR, the fish symbol has survived in amulets and talismans. A second cross, incidentally, formed by the palindromic word TENET as it occurs twice, is hidden in the square itself (Jerphanion, 1938), and it may not be coincidence that the letters *A* and *O* stand at each extremity of this cross (Carcopino, 1953).

Thus a brilliant and satisfactory explanation of the extraordinary SATOR square had finally been evolved. As Jerphanion points out, now one could understand the rapid spread of the square by Christians through the Roman Empire, the popularity of SATOR, and its frequent occurrence in churches. Then, eleven years after Grosser's paper appeared, an Italian discovery reopened the whole question.

Early in 1937 Professor Matteo Della Corte, director of excavations at Pompeii, published two reports stating that he had found

R O T A S

O P E R A

T E N E T

A R E P O

S A T O R

clearly inscribed on a column in that ancient city (Della Corte, 1937 a, b). A colleague had noticed the same square ten years earlier on another building in Pompeii. The unlikely possibility that a practical joker had read the Grosser article and had added a modern *graffito* was ruled out when it was learned that Della Corte had first copied the inscription, found in a new excavation, into his notebook on 5 October 1925, *before* Grosser's article was published.

The Italian announcement raised a serious doubt about Grosser's hypothesis simply because Pompeii had been overwhelmed by Vesuvius in A.D. 79. Could there have been Christians in the doomed city at that early date? If not, how could one accept the German's brilliant explanation?

Jerphanion reviews the evidence and arguments with care. He points out that in A.D. 60 or 61 Paul visited Puteoli (now Pozzuoli), not far from Pompeii, "where we found brethren" (Acts 28:13–14). The latter, of course, were Christians. On the other hand, there is no indication that the Scriptures, including the Lord's Prayer, existed in Latin as early as the first century. They were recorded in Greek, which then was also the language of the early church. The words of the SATOR square are Latin. Also, it is said to be most unlikely that the cross had become a Christian symbol as early as A.D. 79. But to reject the theory that the square was invented by or for a Christian seems to leave the alternative that the crosses and paternosters were due to coincidence, which appears impossible (Carcopino, 1953; Jerphanion, 1938).

The debate is one for specialists, and it continues (Last, 1954). In fact, another explanation has been suggested by Franz Cumont and others. This turns to the Biblical description of the vision of Ezekiel, with its repeated reference to wheels. The Vulgate version (Ezekiel 1:15) employs both *rota* and *opera*.[18] The letter T (tau), it has been suggested, may refer to the protective mark placed "upon the foreheads of the men that sigh" (9:4), and the wheels that "went upon their four sides; and they turned not when they went" (1:17) may mean that if SATOR is read around the periphery of the square, like a wheel with "four sides," the direction of the word is first clockwise and then counterclockwise, as for a wheel which rotates but returns to its original position. According to this hypothesis, the square may have been devised by a Jew inspired by the vivid passage in Ezekiel. Subsequently the square could have been carried to Pompeii by others of his faith. Jerphanion says that there were many Jews in Pompeii and that they made their wall markings in Latin. Finally, of course, the square might have been appropriated by Christians (Carcopino, 1953; Jerphanion, 1938).

Again one must admire an ingenious hypothesis. But somehow it lacks the conviction of Grosser's explanation. Clearly, the last word is yet to be said; the SATOR square, which has puzzled scholars since the Middle Ages, puzzles us still.

18. *Aspectus rotarum et opus earum quasi visio maris . . . et aspectus earum et opera quasi sit rota in medio rotae* (the appearance of the wheels and their work was like a vision of the sea . . . and their appearance and works was, as it were, like a wheel in the middle of a wheel) (Ezek. 1:16; Jerphanion, 1938). See also Ezek. 1:15–21; 10:2,6,9–19; 11:22.

7

The Veil of
Good Fortune

Some children are "born lucky." Infrequently a baby comes into the world with a thin, translucent tissue, a fragment of the amniotic membrane, covering its head (Fig. 5). The remnant is known as a *caul*. The modern obstetrician quickly removes and dis-

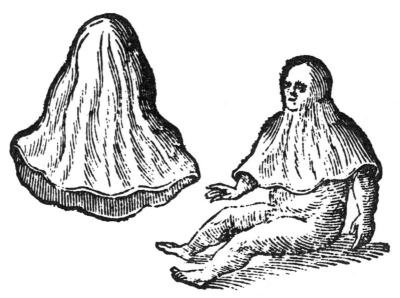

Fig. 5. Infant with caul, from Cornelius Gemma, *De naturae divinis characterismis,* 1575. As in many early pictures of infants, the bodily proportions are those of the adult.

cards the membrane (it may interfere with the infant's efforts to begin respiration). His professional predecessors, the physicians and mid-wives of earlier centuries, would have preserved it, for strong magic and strange beliefs were once related to the caul.

In countries all over the world there developed the curious idea that a caul would bring fame and fortune to its owner. The superstition is at least as old as the ancient Chaldeans (Rubin, 1888) and has not yet disappeared. Aelius Lampridius, a classical historian, related that Emperor Antonius Diadumenianus or Diadematus (b. A.D. 208) was so called because at birth his head was encircled with a fillet (*diadema*), twisted like a bowstring and so strong it could not be broken. One supposes that the caul in this case had been rolled into a band. Although the possession of the fillet was expected to bring him good luck, Diadumenianus was assassinated as a youth.[1] Many years later (1575) Cornelius Gemma, a physician who scorned belief in the powers of the caul, described it quaintly as:

> nothing other than the remnant of another membrane, much softer than the amnion, but nevertheless more solid, bound with a purple border or fringe, and wrapped around the whole head down to the umbilicus, not without great danger to the baby unless the membrane was removed as quickly as possible; thus I myself have observed it in my first-born son who came helmeted [*galeatus*] into the world.

And R. Willis (1639), writing his memoirs, relates:

> ther was one special remarkable thing concerning my self, who being my parents first son, but their second child (they having a daughter before me) when I came into the world, my head, face, and foreparts of the body were all covered over with a thin kell or skin, wrought like an artificiall veile; as also my eldest son being likewise my second childe was borne with the like extraordinary covering: our Midwives and Gossips holding such children as come so veyled into the world to be very fortunate (as they call it).

The beneficent effect of the caul was sometimes regarded as extending to the offspring of the original owner, but, according to a superstition of the Middle Ages and later, this effect would be lost if the caul were given away or sold outside the family (Anon., 1899). On 20 May

1. Drelincurtius (1727), F.C.H. (1857), Magie (1924), Smith (1849).

1658 the will of "Sir John Offley, Knight of Madely Manor, Stafford-shire" was probated. The document included the following bequest:

> Item, I will and devise one Jewell done all in Gold enammelled, wherein there is a Caul that covered my face and shoulders when I first came into the world, the use thereof to my loving Daughter the Lady Elizabeth Jenny, so long as she shall live; and after her decease the use likewise thereof to her son, Offley Jenny, during his natural life; and after his decease to my own right heirs male for ever; and so from Heir to Heir, to be left so long as it shall please God of his Goodness to continue any Heir Male of my name, desiring the same Jewell be not concealed nor sold by any of them. [Cestriensis, 1853]

One notes that the bequest refers not only to the possession but also to the "use" of this curious heirloom.

Lemnius discussed the caul in his *De Miraculis Occultis Naturae,* first published in 1559. A 1658 edition of this work in English, includes the chapter heading: "Of the Helmets of Children newly born, or of the thin and soft caul, wherewith the face is covered as with a vizard, or covering, when they come first into the world." He quotes

> old Wives [who] speak many fabulous things, and fright or cheer the childbearing woman. If this cover be black they speak as from an Oracle (when as they do but dote, and know not what they say) that such children will suffer many sad accidents, and that many misfortunes hang over their heads, and that ill spirits will haunt them, and shall be vexed with dreams and night visions, unless this be broken and given in drink, which against my will many have done to the great hurt of the child. But if this cover be red, or the skin that is fast to the crown of the head, they prophesie that he will be a notable child, and shall have great successe in all his affairs.

In nineteenth-century Scotland and England a mother was advised to preserve her son's caul with care; it would stay white and dry so long as he lived but would turn black and wet at his death. Furthermore, if the caul were lost, the son would be a wanderer and die violently.[2] A similar idea, no doubt imported from Europe, was held by

2. Hastings (1910), J.T.F. (1899), Leach (1949), Nicholson (1890), Rorie(1904), Sykes (1886).

southern Negroes in the United States (Leach, 1949; Puckett, 1926). Closely related was amniomancy, the practice of foretelling the future by inspection of the caul.[3] Since dried cauls apparently did change in appearance, possibly owing to the weather, a superstitious owner might on occasion have an unpleasant shock (Henderson, 1866).

In Herzegovina, a part of Yugoslavia, it was thought that a baby born with a black caul would grow up to become a witch or sorcerer and after death a vampire unless, on the first night after the birth, a woman carried the caul to the rooftop and announced: "A child was born at our house in a bloody shirt." Elsewhere in Yugoslavia the midwife carried the newborn baby itself to the threshold and announced three times that a real baby had been born—not a witch or sorcerer. Whether these procedures were regarded as charms or simply as attempts to prevent superstitious rumors among the neighbors is not reported. In Romania the child with a caul was dreaded because he had the evil eye (Ploss et al., 1935; Seligmann, 1922).

"Shirt" was only one of a great number of synonyms for the caul. Andrews (1947) and others have shown that semantic changes often involve a shift in meaning from the general to the specific. Certainly several terms which originally identified the entire amnion came later to signify only *caul*. Caul itself, on the other hand, and also *kell* were sometimes used as synonyms of amnion. (Caul, in addition, could mean a net, the web of a spider, the base of a wig, a woman's cap, and any of several anatomical investing layers.)

In different lands the same ideas suggested themselves repeatedly in the fanciful terms appropriated to identify the caul. The Latin name [4] *membrana agnina* (lambskin) was equivalent to *membrane agnelette* (French) and *Schafhäutlein* (German). (The Greek work *amnion*, incidentally, is the diminutive of *amnos*, lamb.) Some other, more or less equivalent terms were:

galea (Latin: helmet); *Helm, Helmlein, Barnhelm, Knabenhelm, Knableinhelm* (German, Dutch: helmet, little helmet, crib helmet, little boy's helmet)
pileus, pileolus (Latin: a close-fitting cap like a skull cap); *Haube, Häublein, Hauberl, Hütlin, Glückshaube, Wasserhaube, Wehmutter-*

3. Bargheer (1931), Buschan (1941), Leach (1949), Spence (1920).
4. It is important to remember that Latin was the language of medicine and science until the end of the seventeenth century and beyond. Thus it is not surprising that some of the Latin medical terms designating a caul were translated literally into various European languages.

Häublein, Sturmhaub, Mägdlein-Haube, Westerhut, Westerhaube (German: cap, little cap, lucky cap, water cap, midwife's cap, storm hat, servant's cap, christening cap); *silly hood, silly how, sely how, haly how, lucky hood* (English, Scottish: lucky or holy cap or hood); *calotte* (French: cap)

Kindesnetzlein (German: little child's net); *coiffe, coëffe, petite toile* (French: veil, little cloth); *veil* (English)

involucrum (Latin: wrapper, cover); *Kinderbälglein, Kindbälgel* (German: little child's wrapper or bag); *súpot* (Tagalog, bag, paper bag)

amiculum (Latin: cloak); *sigurkufl* (Icelandic: coat, cape)

indumentum, (pellis) secundina (Latin: mask, second skin); *mask* (English)

indusium, vestis (Latin: shirt, undergarment); *Hemd, Hemdlein, Hemmetlin, Kleidchen, Geburtshemdlein, Glückshemd, Westerhemd, Westerwat* (German: shirt, little shirt, little birth shirt, lucky shirt, christening shirt, christening garment); *kosuljica* (Serbian: little shirt)

Muttergotteshemdlein, camicia della Madonna (German, Italian: Virgin's shift)[5]

The list could be extended, but this is enough to emphasize how the same ideas recurred—helmet, cap, veil, mask, undergarment—all of them suggesting something which, like the caul, fits closely to the body.

As would be expected, literary references to the caul are not uncommon. The *Oxford Dictionary* gives examples dated as early as 1547 (Murray, 1893). *Kell,* a variant of the term, had appeared in print by 1530. Subsequently, the caul was alluded to in English plays, poetry, and novels.[6] Hans Sachs, German poet and shoemaker, and the tower-

5. Adelmann (1942), Bächtold-Stäubli (1930), Bargheer (1931), Bartels (1900), Brand (1810), Brissaud (1892), Browne (1646), Galen (1550), Grimm (1883), Grimm and Grimm (1873), Haller (1775), Hansemann (1914), Hazlitt (1870), Hovorka and Kronfeld (1908), Hyrtl (1884), Lewis and Short (1907), Pettigrew (1844), Ploss et al. (1935), Rorie (1904), Rubin (1888), Rueff (1554), Spigelius (1626), Temesváry (1900), Weissbart (1906), Wirsung (1568).

6. The plays include Ben Jonson's *The Alchemists* (I, 1,327), George Digby's *Elvira* (V), and Thomas Morton's more recent *Secrets Worth Knowing* (I, 1). Thomas Hood, an unquenchable punster, wrote of the mariner who drowned even though he carried an amulet:

> Heaven never heard his cry, nor did
> The ocean heed his caul.
>
> (1857, *The Sea-Spell*)

"I was born with a caul," said David Copperfield (Dickens, 1850) and the hero of at least one other nineteenth-century novel (Coster, 1893) had the same good fortune.

ing Leonardo da Vinci are both said to have been born with cauls (O'Malley and Saunders, 1952; Rubin, 1888).

Because of the pronunciation and meaning of *cowl*, it has been suggested that this word is cognate with *caul* and the related Scottish *kell* (Murray, 1893; Timbs, 1873). A fancied similarity of the monk's cowl to the caul is also said to be the basis of the belief that a child born with a caul was destined by Providence for the monastery or convent (Brissaud, 1892). In Austria it was expected that a boy would become an archbishop if he carried his caul in his clothing (Hovorka and Kronfeld, 1908), and, according to one story, a Chinese youngster who was born with a caul grew up to become a saint and a Buddha (Tsay, 1918). The chronicler Holinshed reports that in the time of King John (thirteenth century) it was the custom to bury the nobility in monks' cowls, and it has been suggested that such cowls were regarded as protective amulets like the caul, which also covered the head (B.B., 1852; Timbs, 1873). This seems an ingenious but unlikely idea. St. Chrysostom (347?–407) is said to have preached several sermons against the caul superstition and to have criticized in particular a clergyman, one Praetus or Protus, who bought a "veil" from a midwife to ensure good fortune (Grose, 1811; Migne, 1856). Theodore Balsamo, a Church Father who died in 1180, tells of a similar incident involving a layman (1865; Migne, 1856):

> A certain prefect of Hosius, accused of this sort of thing, was arrested when caught in the act of carrying in his bosom the *indumentum* of a newborn infant, and said this had been given to him by a certain woman for the purpose of turning away and stopping up the mouths of those who tried to speak against him. Whence he was the subject of condemnation.

There is a tale about "a certain jealous fellow" who was so suspicious of his wife and an innocent Franciscan monk that she dared not attend church. When her son was born, he had a caul on his head.

> The happy woman, . . . hoping to increase [her husband's] joy at the birth of the little one, said that he had come into the light with the appearance of a friar. Many women, as you know, think it is a good omen for an infant to be born with a caul. When that miserable jealous fellow heard from her of the cowled infant, he at once thought it had been fathered by the Franciscan. His patience thereupon at an end, seizing the child from her he sought to dash it

on the ground but was prevented by the bystanders. [Guainerius, 1500]

Notes and Queries, that extraordinary repository of antiquarian and other information, offers a quotation from a British newspaper, the Leeds *Mercury,* for 14 September 1889. A laborer's wife bore a son on whose head was a caul. The membrane was laid aside unnoticed for several hours. Then someone picked it up and was astounded to see the words "British and Foreign Bible Society" clearly impressed in the now dry caul. Friends and neighbors flocked to see what some of them considered a miracle. The physician who delivered the baby was skeptical, and soon found that the moist caul when first removed had somehow been laid on the cover of a Bible on which the words were impressed. But this prosaic explanation was rejected by some local enthusiasts, who remained convinced that the baby was a born missionary with a great future (M.P., 1889).

In Iceland, in the Kentucky mountains, and in the islands near New Guinea, the fortunate person who wore a caul at birth was held to have powers of clairvoyance;[7] the Dutch, as well as North American and West Indian Negroes, were sure that he could see and talk with ghosts.[8] The caul was also a protection against sorcery, evil spirits, and demons, and against the dread possibility that a witch or fairy would carry off the baby and leave in its place her ugly offspring, a changeling.[9] In time of war, the caul was variously regarded as a protection against prolonged military service (Germany) and injury in battle (Netherlands Indies) or as a guarantee of success in warfare (Maoris of New Zealand).[10]

Many people were convinced that the caul should be either preserved or carefully disposed of at childbirth. There was a widespread belief that in the caul resided the child's guardian spirit or "life token"[11] and that careless treatment of the membrane would deprive the child of an important protective influence. In Iceland the caul was usually buried by the midwife under the threshold over which the mother would later pass; Hastings suggests that this may have been done so

7. Bartels (1900), Frazer (1935), Moorehouse (1898), Pickin (1909), Thomas and Thomas (1920).
8. Babcock (1888), Beckwith (1929), Hastings (1910), Leach (1949), Puckett (1926).
9. Bartels (1900), Dyer (1881), Leach (1949).
10. Goldie (1904), Ploss (1872), Riedel (1886b, n.d.), Temesváry (1900).
11. Bartels (1900), Grimm (1883), Hastings (1910), Hovorka and Kronfeld (1908), Leach (1949), MacCulloch (1930), Ploss (1872).

that if the child died, its spirit could return to the mother and be born again. The amnion would be entered by evil spirits if discarded in the open, while the baby would lose its soul if the membrane were burned.[12] In Russia loss of the caul meant trouble ahead for the infant (Hastings, 1910). In other lands, great misfortune or even death awaited him whose caul was lost, torn, or buried.[13] A Belgian child would be lucky if the caul was preserved or buried in a field, unlucky if the remnant was burned or thrown onto the trash heap (Ploss, 1872). The mother of Vesalius, the great Belgian anatomist, held such a belief (O'Malley, 1964). Vesalius himself makes passing reference in the *Fabrica* (1543) to preservation of the caul by ignorant people, adding that both midwives and "secret philosophers" greatly coveted it. Quite clearly, however, he himself spurned the superstition.

The "veil" was, of course, frequently worn in the clothing or carried as an amulet.[14] It might even be eaten by the owner in an egg dish. In the islands near New Guinea, a child was washed with water in which the caul had been steeped and was later fed the powdered caul to free him from its concomitant clairvoyance, which evidently was not always regarded as an asset. On the other hand, in Pomerania it was believed that if the caul was burned to a powder and then given to the baby with its milk, the child would become a vampire or a butcher-bird. In Ireland the caul of a farm animal was considered a harbinger of good luck and was carefully thrown over a beam of the house.[15]

Sometimes the midwife stole the caul so that she could give it to another child or sell it to a witch.[16] Witches were reported to prize cauls highly as potent aids in evildoing. The *Journal de L'Estoile pour le Regne de Henri IV,* a colorful account of daily events in Paris in the sixteenth century, tells how two priests who were also practitioners of witchcraft battled for a caul in a church on 21 October 1596. It seems that one, *le sorcier,* forgot to take his caul with him when he left the altar. The other, finding the caul, refused to return it, whereupon a noisy quarrel followed *avec grande scandale de tout le peuple.* The finder of the caul succeeded in retaining it, but was promptly accused

12. Bartels (1900), Buschan (1941), Hastings (1910), Hovorka and Kronfeld (1908).
13. Leach (1949), Sykes (1886), Wuttke (1900).
14. Abbott (1903), Grimm (1883), Grimm and Grimm (1873), Hastings (1910), Hovorka and Kronfeld (1908), Pickin (1909), Ploss et al. (1935), Weissbart (1906).
15. Frazer (1935), Hovorka and Kronfeld (1908), Jahn (1886), Temesváry (1900), Weissbart (1906), Wilde (1849).
16. Bartholin (1677), Chanter (1923), Grose (1811), Ploss (1872), Puckett (1926), Wuttke (1900).

of sorcery and thrown into prison. He escaped with the help of his friends and proceeded to take his revenge on his colleague (Lefèvre, 1948). That possession of a caul was thought to be worth such a scandalous episode clearly illustrates the strength of the superstition at that time.

This account may have further significance, since it is known that cauls were sometimes baptized. The infamous sorcerer-priest perhaps had brought the caul to the altar for that purpose. The Church of course viewed as a sacrilege the baptism

> of dead flesh, be it of man or animal, as do those who preserve the membrane in which their children come into the world; they baptize it and anoint it with holy oils, as if they confirmed it, in order later to make horrible witchcraft with it. Saint Bernard of Siena speaks of this execrable baptism. [LeBrun and Thiers, 1733]

It seems probable that baptism of the caul began quite innocently as an outgrowth of the superstition, previously mentioned, that this membrane was a part of the baby or contained its spirit. Thus German midwives smuggled the caul into the baptismal chest, and in Hungary a sack containing the caul was placed under the baby's head at the christening.[17] In this way the "veil" was also blessed at the ceremony.

There are numerous records that the caul was employed in witchcraft. In 1617 Louise Bourgeois, famed midwife to the court of France, in a textbook of obstetrics intended for her daughter spoke her mind on the ethics of midwifery and included a specific warning about the caul (p. 206): *Ne retenes jamais la membrane amnios (dit la coiffe de l'enfant, de laquelle aucuns enfans viennent couuerts la test & les epaules) d'autant que les sourciers s'en séruent* (never preserve the caul, lest it be used by sorcerers). And Thomas Bartholin (1677), the Danish physician, tells darkly how midwives "preserve such a helmet of a little boy or the small cap of a little girl to take care of sundry needs." One such was as an ingredient in a love potion or "philter." Burton's *Anatomy of Melancholy* (Democritus, 1638) specifies for such a brew a swallow's heart, "dust of a Doves heart," vipers' tongues, the brains of donkeys, the membrane (caul?) of a horse, "the cloak with which infants are wrapped when they are born," rope with which

17. Buschan (1941), Hovorka and Kronfeld (1908), Knortz (1909).

a man was hanged, and a stone from the nest of an eagle. Other cases of outright witchcraft involving cauls could be added.[18]

Brissaud (1892) tells how maidens would ask the women assisting in a delivery to save the caul, "believing that if this powder were given to a man, he would at once fall in love with a maiden." In Germany a young man carried his caul with him to aid him in winning the affection of a girl (Ploss, 1872). In the southern Slavic countries a girl wore her caul as a love charm; if she then touched the skin of a man, he would instantly be attracted to her (Hovorka and Kronfeld, 1908). Lean (1903) reports that a Scottish expression, *rowed in his mother's sark-tail,* that is, wrapped in his mother's shift, is associated with the belief that an adult who had been so protected as a baby would be successful in his love affairs. Lean suggests that all this related to the superstition about the caul as a love charm.

The membrane was even valuable to the farmer. On the Island of Timor he used it as an amulet to save a failing rice crop (Frazer, 1935). The White Russian farmer counted on the caul to ensure healthy cattle and good harvests (Bartels, 1907).

The "veil" was widely believed to make its owner eloquent. A biography of Antonius Diadumenianus, the Roman emperor who was born with a caul, says that midwives sold cauls for large sums to credulous lawyers who sought eloquence in court (Drelincurtius, 1727; F.C.H., 1857). The superstition was strong in Iceland, England, Denmark, and elsewhere.[19] The similarity, too, between the lawyer's coif and the caul has not escaped notice (Hazlitt, 1905; Snell, 1911).

In medicine the caul was valued highly as a remedy, both general and specific (Brand, 1810). From Norse mythology came the belief that if the caul had been dedicated to the Norns, giant goddesses who held men's fates in their hands, childbirth would be easy (Ploss, 1884). In Denmark it was thought that a woman who crept under a foal's caul stretched on sticks would have a painless labor, but as a penalty her sons would become werewolves and her daughters night hags (M.G.W.P., 1897). Medicines made from the caul could cure a variety of sicknesses in the owner.[20] An old remedy for malaria included snails, egg white, laurel berries, powder from a burned piece of shirt,

18. LeBrun and Thiers (1733), Spindler (1691), Valentini (1722).
19. Bartels (1900), Bartholin (1676), Hovorka and Kronfeld (1908), Snell (1911), Wuttke (1900).
20. Bartholin (1676), Beckwith (1929), Crawley (1902), Frazer (1935).

rust from a coffin nail, a pinch of burned and powdered human bone, *and* a powdered caul (Hovorka and Kronfeld, 1908). Unfortunately, the rationale for this masterpiece is not stated. In Dalmatia, the caul was placed under the owner's head when he lay on his death bed so that his passing would be easy (Ploss et al., 1927).

Many physicians were skeptical about the alleged powers of the membrane. Paré (Johnson, 1665) concluded that in a difficult birth the amnion would always be stripped away from the infant, just as "the Snake or Adder when she should cast her skin thereby to renew her skin, creepeth through some strait or narrow passage." Mauriceau, in his textbook of obstetrics (1775) rejects the superstition and dryly remarks that children with cauls "may be said to be fortunate, for having been born so easily; and the Mother also for having been so speedily delivered; for the difficult Labours, Children are never born with such Caps, because being tormented and pressed in the Passage, these Membranes are broken and remain there."

Beliefs about the caul were recognized by Sir Thomas Browne (1646):

> Great conceits are raised of the membranous covering, commonly called the Silly-how, that sometimes is found upon the heads of children upon their birth; and is therefore preserved with great care, not only as medical in diseases, but effectual in success, concerning the Infant and others; which is surely no more than a continued superstition.

Van der Spiegel, a Belgian anatomist, described how the amniotic membrane may in childbirth "be draped partly or completely around the head, so that in the male it may be called a helmet by the German obstetricians, or in the female, as the Italians put it, a fillet or shirt." He suggested that it is ridiculous to attach supernatural significance to a phenomenon which can be readily explained (Spigelius, 1626). Joubert (1578) was equally contemptuous: "It is true that if he [one who carries a caul for protection] falls off a horse and breaks his legs, the pieces [of the caul] will be found in his boots, if he has any. What nonsense!" Charles Drelincourt (1633-97), another physician, wrote *De foetum pileolo sive galea* [*On the Little Cap or Helmet of Fetuses*] (1727). Unfortunately, his rather extended discussion consisted largely of harsh sarcasm directed at the ideas of some of his colleagues regarding the caul. Drelincourt made it clear that he too rejected any idea of the membrane's power to bring good fortune. Thomas Bartholin (1677) and Jane Sharp (1671) said they had known of unlucky children who were born with cauls and lucky children who were born without them. And at least one Swiss physician wrote scornfully about the superstition (Muralt, 1697).

In the eighteenth century, Thiers, in his interesting *Traité des superstitions* (1741), quoted the French proverb that the happy man was born with a veil (*est né coëffé*) and expressed the opinion that any advantage to one who wears the caul as a charm could come only with the help of the devil. Haller, the Swiss physiologist, made passing reference in his *Physiologie* (1774) to the caul as a supposed sign of good luck. Spindler (1691), a physician, said that he had never heard of a caul worn as a charm bringing good luck, but then told of a male patient who ascribed his impotence to the fact that his wife wore such a charm (i.e. the caul could have an evil influence).

If the caul could ensure well-being, it could also ward off disaster and danger.[21] Coal miners carried cauls to prevent the explosion of fire damp (Brissaud, 1892), and there is a relatively recent report of an English farmer who ascribed his own good health and that of his two sons, then fighting in World War I, to the fact that each of them carried the caul of a lamb born in the farmer's flock (Weeks, 1923). This would seem to be simply an extension of the idea of the protective influence of the human caul. (Recollect that both the human amnion and the caul proper were sometimes compared to lambskin.)

One of the most widespread of all the caul superstitions was that it would protect against drowning. Very likely, as has been suggested (Fairfax-Blakeborough, 1923; McKenzie, 1927), the idea sprang from the fact that the fetus does not drown in the fluid enclosed by the amnion, of which the caul is a fragment. In the Middle Ages a caul was considered a protection against the demons who caused storms at sea, and for centuries the "veil" has been carried by sailors to save them from shipwreck and drowning.[22] In one of Captain Marryat's novels, a bundle dropped into the Thames does not sink because, of course, it contains a caul (Philips, 1923). The inventions of novelists, however, were exceeded by fact. A contributor to *Frank Leslie's Illustrated Newspaper* (Gardner, 1870) reports of a renowned orator and critic:

21. Bartels (1900), Glück (1894), Grgjič-Bjelokosic (1899).
22. Dyer (1881), Trachtenberg (1939), Trevelyan (1909).

a man who had a half-dozen languages at his tongue's end, a fine conversationalist, a distinguished writer and scholar . . . and one who would be supposed to have considerable reason and thought —that this individual came to this country safely under the protection of a "caul"; that he sent it back again as an aegis to his family, who followed him, and repeatedly lent it to friends crossing and recrossing the ocean.

Other testimony appeared in *Notes and Queries* (J.T.F., 1899). A baby born with a caul was protected so effectively "that when his mother tried to bathe him he sat on the surface of the water, and if forced down, came up again like a cork." An instance of miraculous preservation from drowning of a man born with a caul has been alleged very recently (Baines, 1950); the superstition still exists in the twentieth century (Fairfax-Blakeborough, 1923; Hole, 1957).

Cauls were occasionally advertised for sale in the newspapers and also in shops. Readers of the *London Morning Post* for 21 August 1779 noted:

> To the gentlemen of the Navy, and others going long voyages to sea. To be disposed of, a child's caul. Enquire at the Bartlett Buildings Coffee House in Holborn. N.B. To avoid unnecessary trouble the price is Twenty Guineas.

By 1799 the price paid by British sailors had reached thirty guineas. These were the days of the Napoleonic Wars and great sea battles. Perhaps the naval outlook was somewhat better early in 1813, for the *London Times* of 20 February in that year revealed a lower asking price:

> A child's caul to be sold, in the highest perfection. Enquire at No. 2, Church Street, Minories. To prevent trouble, price of £12.

Two more cauls were advertised without prices a week later in the same paper. The going rate in 1815 was twelve guineas; the *Times* of 8 December 1819 offered a caul at fifteen guineas.[23]

An advertisement in the same paper for 1820 did not name a price, but in 1835 a *Times* insert read: "A Child's Caul to be disposed of, a well known preservative against drowning, &c., price 10 guineas." On 8 May 1848 the newspaper carried the following:

23. Ackermann (1923), Fairfax-Blakeborough (1923), Hazlitt (1905), Kanner (1931), St. Swithin (1915).

A child's caul. Price six guineas. Apply at the bar of the Tower Shades, corner of Tower Street. The above article, for which fifteen pounds was originally paid, was afloat with its late owner thirty years in all perils of a seaman's life, and the owner died at last in the place of his birth.

The *Western Daily News* of Plymouth offered a caul for five guineas on 9 February 1867, while the asking price in the *Liverpool Mercury* in 1873 was from two guineas down to thirty shillings. There was a caul advertisement in a Liverpool paper in 1891. It is instructive to realize that London, Plymouth, and Liverpool are all major ports, as is Bristol, where the *Times and Mirror* for 30 September 1874 displayed on its front page: "TO SEA CAPTAINS. For sale, a Child's Caul in perfect condition. £5. O.H., Bath Post Office. 2554." [24]

The market must have been unsteady in 1895. Advertisers from Hull and Derbyshire in the *Bazaar* of 15 and 22 March suggested "5 *l.* [pounds] or offers" and "1 *l.* or offers," while three insertions in the *Star* for 20 December asked for £3 or offers. That eminent medical journal, *The Lancet,* noted on page 137 of its issue of 14 January 1899 that cauls were displayed for sale in shop windows near the Liverpool and London docks. A man in Berkshire advertised a caul for sale in the *Globe* of 24 July 1903 ("no reasonable offer refused"), and £3 was asked in the *Daily Express* of 23 August 1904 for a male caul. In the last years before World War I cauls were bought for a few shillings. [25]

But then prices rose. As the deadly submarine attacks occurred in 1915, superstitious sailors naturally made new demands for cauls. An interested observer, who not long before the war had purchased them near the London Docks for eighteen pence apiece, found that by August 1915 submarine warfare had pushed the price up to two pounds. Elsewhere during the great conflict, prices of from three guineas to five pounds were noted. As with many other commodities, ensuing years have not lowered the cost. In 1954 a British midwife tried to buy a caul for ten pounds, wishing to give it to a sailor. The offer was declined by the mother, who chose instead to ensure the good fortune of her own son by retaining the veil with which he had been born. [26]

24. Jones (1880), Kanner (1931), Malins (1874), Moore (1891).
25. Ackermann (1923), Anon. (1899), Fairfax-Blakeborough (1923), J.T.F. (1904), M.G.W.P. (1897), St. Swithin (1915).
26. Ackermann (1923), Chanter (1923), Fairfax-Blakeborough (1923), Hole (1957), Lovett (1925), St. Swithin (1915).

Sometimes confused with the caul of a horse was the *hippomanes,* an object well known to classical writers. The caul and the hippomanes in fact are not the same thing, but both words identify unusual remnants of the fetal membranes. In ancient times and down through the Middle Ages, *hippomanes* (Latin, Greek; French, *hippomane;* German, *Füllengift, Fohlenmilz, Fohlenbrot;* etc.) signified variously a poison, a love potion or ingredient thereof, a plant that produces estrus in the mare, estrus itself, the estrous secretion, or particularly a bit of dark flesh said to lie on the forehead of the newborn foal.[27] According to recent interpretations, the hippomanes as last defined is the result of a local accumulation of the secretion from the glands of the pregnant uterus of various ungulates, including the horse, and of at least one primate. The enlarging mass causes in the horse the progressive invagination of the overlying area of chorio-allantoic membrane into the allantoic cavity or, in the lemur, into the yolk sac. When fully formed, the hippomanes consists of a small round or elongate mass of viscous material invested with chorio-allantoic or chorion-yolk sac membrane; the membrane also provides the pedicle connecting the structure to the inner surface of the allantois or yolk sac proper. The sac has recently been referred to as an allantochorionic pouch. Thieke states that the hippomanes may even become detached and lie free in the allantoic cavity between the embryo and its membranes.[28]

One can imagine that a foal might be born with either an amniotic fragment (the equivalent of the human caul) or a true chorio-allantoic hippomanes adhering to its head; presumably such an occurrence inspired the inaccurate classical concept. Aristotle (1910 ed.) describes the growth as black, round, and smaller than a dried fig. The mare, he says, promptly bites off and swallows the hippomanes; if someone steals it (as a love charm) and the mare catches its odor, she becomes frantic. The mass was highly prized as the ingredient of potions. Vergil (1938 ed.) tells how Dido, desperate because Aeneas was going to leave her, asks a witch to cast magic spells. The witch-priestess

> with dishevelled hair three times calls loudly on the hundred gods, Erebus and Chaos and the three-fold Hecate, the triple faces of the

27. Aristotle (1910), Bächtold-Stäubli (1930), Buffon (1753), Clauderus (1685), Collin de Plancy (1826), Columella (1745), Juvenal (1928), Murray (1893), Ovidius Naso (1947), Thieke (1911), Vergilius Maro (1938).
28. Clegg et al. (1954), Hamlett (1935), Hammond (1927), Thieke (1911).

maiden Diana. She had strewn about simulated water of the lake of Avernus, and search is made for luxuriant herbs, cut with brazen sickles in the light of the moon, and having a juice of black poison. She looks too for the hippomanes,[29] snatched from the forehead of the newborn colt to forestall its mother.

In the first century A.D., Lucan, discussing love philters, mentions the hippomanes as a powerful agent. Juvenal and Suetonius both tell how the Empress Caesonia prepared a love potion from the hippomanes for her husband Caligula; the drink, however, drove him mad.[30] Philemon Holland's translation of Pliny (1601) fills in details:

> These foles verily, by report, have growing on their forehead, when they bee newly come into the world, a little blacke thing of the bignesse of a fig, called Hippomanes, and it is thought to have an effectual vertue to procure and win love. The dam hath not so soon foled, but she bites it off, and eats it her selfe: and if it chance that any body preventeth her of it, and catcheth it from her, she will never let the fole sucke her. The very smell and sent thereof, if it be stollen away, will drive them into a fit of rage and madnesse.

Columella in the first century A.D., Aelian and Solinus in the third, Photius in the ninth, and Bartholomew the Englishman in the thirteenth century followed Aristotle closely in their descriptions of the hippomanes. Aelian added that the mare's rage when the *caruncula* is stolen is due to her jealousy of the sorcerers who would make use of the mass in potions for human beings.[31]

After Europe emerged from the Dark Ages, references to the hippomanes again appeared. Barnabe Googe's books on husbandry repeated earlier authority. Porta mentioned the hippomanes in his *Magiae naturalis libri XX* in connection with love potions, as did Wier in a chapter entitled "De veneficis," Castro and Delrio in chapters on philters, and Wecker in the formula for a love potion.[32] It is noteworthy that *veneficus* signified both a sorcerer and a poisoner, just as *veneficium* meant both witchcraft and poisoning. Thomas Shadwell made fun of witchcraft in his play, *The Lancashire Witches*—a love potion is brewed from the "bunch of Flesh from a black Fole's Head."

29. Lit. *amor*, love.
30. Juvenal (1928), Lucanus (1928), Suetonius Tranquillus (1930).
31. Aelianus (1744), Columella (1745), Photius (1621), Solinus (1554), Steele (1893).
32. Castro (1662), Delrio (1608), Googe (1577), Porta (1910), Weckerus (1587), Wierus (1577).

Markham, in his *Cavelarice, or the English Horseman,* in 1607 rejected the hippomanes superstition—

> but for mine own part, having seene so many Mares foale as I have done, and never perceyuing any such observation, I cannot imagine it any other than a fabulouse dreame.

Ruini's book on the horse, another fascinating work, told, as Thieke has pointed out, of a structure which certainly must be the hippomanes, although Ruini did not give it a name. In a horn of the uterus of the pregnant mare, he says, there has been found an unattached mass which is usually lead-colored, egg-shaped, "and about a half-finger thick if the mare has not carried it for long." Ruini believed that this mass was the poisonous residue of the semen. Clauder remarked that "What the hippomanes actually is, and what its proper use may be, has exercised the wits of physicians and philosophers in many ages." He rejected the superstitions, including the idea that prompt removal of the mass ensured that the foal would become a swift racer and the belief of a colleague that the administration of ten grains of dried hippomanes would protect a child against epilepsy.[33]

Agrippa does not seem to question the hippomanes superstitions in his *Three Books of Occult Philosophy* (1651). Learned articles in Bonet's *Medicina septentrionalis* (1686) and Bayle's great dictionary (1741) review the literature on the hippomanes but do not actually give credence to the superstitions. The strange black mass was discussed at length in two theses (Vater; Wedelius) in 1725. A few years later, Daubenton published (1755, 1756) what appear to be the first attempts to investigate the hippomanes in scientific fashion. As a comparative anatomist particularly interested in the horse, he dissected many pregnant mares and repeatedly found gelatinous masses in the uterus between, he says, the allantois and the amnion. He concluded, *Cette expérience prouve clairement que l'hippomanes est un sédiment de la liqueur contenue entre l'allantoïde & l'amnios.* He also suggested that very rarely a colt might be born with a hippomanes bound to its forehead by an amniotic remnant or *calotte,* like the infants *qui naissent coëffés, selon l'expression vulgaire.* He reported finding the hippomanes of the donkey, cow, deer, goat, and ewe.[34]

33. Clauderus (1685), Markham (1607), Ruinus (1603), Shadwell (1691).
34. Agrippa (1651), Bayle (1741), Bonetus (1686), Daubenton (1755, 1756), Vater (1725), Wedelius (1725).

Buffon in his *Histoire naturelle* and Bourgelat and Sind in volumes on veterinary medicine discussed the hippomanes with considerable understanding. Nineteenth-century works on comparative anatomy described the structure less erroneously and in more detail. It remained for Thieke and Hamlett, however, to dispel misunderstanding of the phenomenon by explaining it. The term *hippomanes,* horse madness, itself survives, testimony to a superstition of the days when biology was born.[35]

35. Blumenbach (1827), Bourgelat (1769), Buffon (1753), Chauveau (1873), Hamlett (1935), Sind (1770), Thieke (1911).

8

The Midwife
and the Witch

The profession of midwife was in general a lowly one during the fifteenth, sixteenth, and part of the seventeenth centuries. It is true that women like Louise Bourgeois and Justine Siegemundin made brave efforts to raise the standard of obstetrical practice. But of what use were the sensible admonitions of Bourgeois' *Observations diverses* (1617) to a woman who could neither read the volume nor afford to buy it? The midwife, particularly in rural areas, was often ignorant and superstitious, and seems frequently to have been the victim of degrading tradition; it is no wonder that she sometimes fell into evil ways.

Medicine as practiced was often at a low level; the position of midwifery was even worse, since for lack of teachers there was usually little formal instruction. Sometimes a village woman was chosen to be a midwife chiefly because she herself had borne several children. The dubious skill which she brought to the delivery was a blend of hearsay, empiricism, and superstition. Medicines were often nasty and frequently of little value. The best chance for mother and infant lay in an uncomplicated delivery and a midwife who had the good sense not to interfere much beyond tying off the cord and encouraging the mother to trust in religion and the power of nature.[1] In some areas the midwives were too numerous, and practice was scanty. In France their fees almost always were wretchedly small, and their economic position was

1. Aveling (1872), Eitel (1914), Garrison (1929), Gosset (1909), Hiltprandus (1595), Klein (1902), Lammert (1869), Rösslin (1513), Thilenius (1775). Aveling's history, *English Midwives,* is a most useful source.

then even more miserable than that of the rest of the peasant popula-tion.[2] The social status of the profession was so low in Bavaria that these women were looked down on even by the barber, the knacker, and the executioner; and the midwife's son might be excluded from a trade guild because of his mother's occupation (Eitel, 1914).

Ignorant, unskilled, poverty-stricken, and avoided as she often was, it is small wonder that the midwife could be tempted, in spite of the teachings of the Church, to indulge in superstitious practices or even in witchcraft. If formally accused of the latter, she stood in grave peril of her freedom or her life, but short of this, she could enjoy great if un-savory prestige, a reputation for secret skills, and perhaps an aug-mented income, as well as the delights of the witches' "sabbath." She could, in fact, capitalize on her status in the community, professing the power (for a fee), to cure disease, foretell the future, find lost or stolen property, prepare love potions, and so on, as well as claiming special skills at the bedside of the woman in labor (Raine, 1861). Sev-eral authorities have suggested that the life of the peasant during the Middle Ages and early Renaissance was so harsh and drab, with little hope of succor in the present or salvation in the future, that the inter-mittent pleasures promised to those who swore allegiance to the devil often offered powerful temptation to the weak and discouraged as well as to the daring.[3]

Witchcraft and devil worship had existed quietly in Western Europe for a very long time before ecclesiastical authority took open cog-nizance of the extent to which these heresies had spread. Gradually it was realized that the "old religion" held powerful sway, especially out-side the cities. In the thirteenth and fourteenth centuries, church and state began to take action, and the prosecution of real and alleged witches slowly spread across Europe, acquiring a terrible momentum.[4] In Great Britain, for example, the first execution for witchcraft took place in 1479; by 1735 and 1736, when the criminal laws against witch-

2. Records of fees for British midwives before 1700 are rather scanty. The fees varied greatly. In 1558 6s.8d. was paid to a midwife who traveled from Somersetshire to London for a confinement; 12d. went to a rural midwife in 1610. A record for January 1612 notes: "given to the midwiffe which helpe a cowe that could not calve ij⁵ vjᵈ." Fees for delivery in a town were higher than they were in the country and were also, some-times, adjusted to the financial circumstances of the patient. Alice Dennis, the midwife who twice delivered Queen Anne, received £100 on each occasion. As a comparison, the average fee for the services of an English physician in the latter part of the seventeenth century was about 10s. (Aveling, 1872; Garrison, 1929; Harland, 1856).
3. Hughes (1952), Raine (1861), Notestein (1911).
4. Castiglioni (1946), Chereau (1881), Hughes (1952), Murray (1937), Wright (1843), Zilboorg (1935).

craft were repealed, approximately 30,000 people had been put to death for this offense. Remy indicated that in the Lorraine section of France about 900 persons were executed for witchcraft in the fifteen years be-

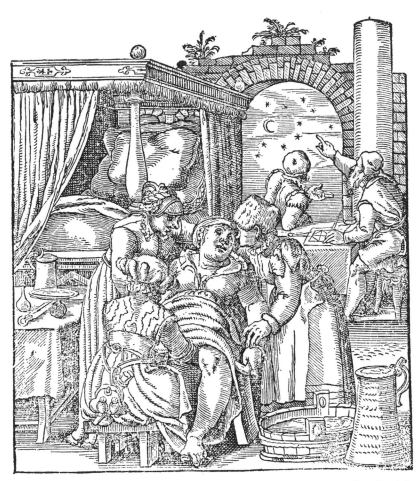

Fig. 6. A delivery room scene from Jacob Rueff's *De conceptu et generatione hominis,* published in Frankfurt in 1580. The woman in labor grips the handles of the birth stool on which she sits, facing the midwife. Two assistants comfort and support the patient. On the table are string and scissors for tying and cutting the cord, and nearby is a tub of water for washing the baby. At the window an astrologer studies the relations of the planets so that he can cast the infant's horoscope. The bed is rather sumptuous, but the patient's well-separated great toe suggests that she seldom wears shoes and hence is a peasant.

fore he published his *Demonolatrie* in 1595.[5] In each of the waves of repression which mounted from time to time, accusations of witchcraft increased. Many of the charges were false, and many "confessions" were extracted by threats, harsh treatment, and torture.[6] But ecclesiastical authority, civil government, and the laity believed in the reality of witchcraft, and here and there it was practiced and the rites of the witches quietly but undoubtedly were performed (Chereau, 1881). To the educated and ignorant alike, the powers of evil and forces of good were seen locked in earthly combat for the possession of men's souls. Each man must align himself with one side or the other.

The repression of witchcraft had the support of the highest authorities. In England, a statute of the realm dating from 1541 (33 Hen. VIII. cap. 8) penalized many acts of witchcraft. The law was repealed in 1547 (1 Edw. VI. cap. 12) but was restored five years later (5 Eliz. cap. 16), citing many offenses which had occurred in the interim. James I considered himself an expert on sorcery. He was so incensed by Reginald Scot's courageous questioning, in his *Discoverie of Witchcraft* (1930 ed.), of popular beliefs about magic and its practitioners that the King not only wrote his own *Daemonologie* in 1597 (when he was still James VI of Scotland) to set the record straight but saw to it that all available copies of Scot's book were burned (Craig, 1932). (A few survived.) A law enacted by the King in 1603 (Jac. I. cap. 12) made many acts of witchcraft felonies and increased the severity of the penalties:

5. Remy (1930), Rogers (1869), Warden (1938).
6. Torture was barred by English common law, but nevertheless was used officially in that country, as it was also in Scotland and on the Continent. Even when the authorities did not take advantage of the horrible devices and skills of the torturer, enforced sleeplessness and appalling prison conditions could be very effective in persuading a prisoner to talk. Sir George Mackenzie, an eminent Scottish legal authority, remarked in 1678, "These poor creatures when they are defamed become so confounded with fear, and the closse Prison in which they are kept, and so starved for want of meat and sleep (either of which wants is enough to disorder the strongest reason) that hardly wiser and more serious people than they would escape distraction. . . .

"Most of these poor creatures are tortur'd by their keepers, who being perswaded they do God good service, think it their duty to vex and torment poor Prisoners."

Sir William Blackstone, commenting on the English witchcraft laws repealed in 1736, says, "These acts continued in force until lately, to the terror of all antient females in the kingdom; and many poor wretches were sacrificed thereby to the prejudice of their neighbours, and their own illusions; not a few having, by some means or other, confessed the fact at the gallows" (Blackstone, 1769; Warden, 1938). However, a good many other witches are believed to have testified quite willingly. The confessions referred to by Blackstone probably were spoken voluntarily just before execution by the victims to clear their consciences; certainly it was too late for legal exculpation. There are a good many eyewitness accounts of such confessions.

If any pson [person] or persons . . . shall use practice or exercise
any Invocation or Conjuration of any evill and wicked Spirit, or
shall consult covenant with entertaine employ feed or rewarde any
evill and wicked Spirit to or for any intent or purpose . . . or shall
use practice or exercise any Witchcraft Inchantement Charme or
Sorcerie, wherebie any pson shalbe killed destroyed wasted consumed pined or lamed in his or her bodie, or any parte thereof; that
then everie such Offendor or Offendors, their Ayders, Abettors and
Counsellors, being of any of the saide Offences dulie and lawfullie
convicted and attainted, shall suffer pains of deathe as a Felon or
Felons, and shall loose the priviledge and benefit of Cleargie and
Sanctuarie.[7]

The Church had long since taken an implacable stand. Pope Innocent VIII denounced witchcraft in his Bull of 1484 (Thompson,
1929). Two Dominican inquisitors, Sprenger and Kraemer, in 1489
published the *Malleus maleficarum*, a grim textbook even for those
harsh days, of detailed directions for the detection, conviction, and
punishment of witches and sorcerers. In the next two hundred years
this work went through at least nineteen editions (Summers, 1928;
Zilboorg, 1935). In view of the opposition of church and state to
witchcraft and of the terrible penalties imposed on convicted offenders,
it is remarkable that anyone deliberately practiced the black arts.[8] Great
crowds attended some of the "sabbaths" at which the devil was wor-
shipped. In earlier times members of the Christian clergy were involved (Murray, 1937), a fact which accounts in part for the vigor
with which the Church sought to root out this heresy.

What was a witch? Murray (1937) quotes the definition of Lord
Coke (1552–1634), an English jurist: "a person who hath conference
with the Devil to consult him or to do some act," a description which
echoes that of Jean Bodin (Castiglioni, 1946). Sir George Mackenzie
has illustrated the combination of biblical authority[9] and circular reasoning that convinced many people about witches: "That there are
Witches, Divines cannot doubt, since the Word of God hath ordain'd
that no Witch shall live, nor Lawyers in *Scotland,* seeing our Law

7. Anon. (1817), Harland (1864), Mackenzie (1678).
8. According to Margaret Murray, a leading modern authority, witchcraft existed as a
pagan religion in England until the eighteenth century and survived until recently in
Italy and France.
9. Exod. 22:18; Deut. 18:10–11, I Sam. 15:23, Gal. 5:20.

ordains it to be punished with death" (1678). The argument died hard. In 1773 Sir William Blackstone wrote:

> To deny the possibility, nay, actual existence of witchcraft and sorcery is at once flatly to contradict the revealed word of God, in various passages both of the old and new testament: and the thing itself is a truth to which every nation in the world hath in its turn borne testimony, by either examples seemingly well attested, or prohibitory laws, which at least suppose the possibility of commerce with evil spirits.

After some examination of the problem, Blackstone suggests: "Wherefore it seems to be the most eligible way to conclude, with an ingenious writer of our own, that in general there has been such a thing as witchcraft; though one cannot give credit to any particular modern instance of it." [10] Very few would now accept the possibility of an actual compact or contact with the powers of evil. We can instead subscribe to the definition, supported by Webster, of a witch as an individual who was *believed* to be in league with the devil and to practice black magic (Neilson, 1944). By this criterion there were witches aplenty.

The question that next arises is, to what extent were midwives actually involved in witchcraft? Certainly they were accused of this offense. The *Malleus maleficarum* (Summers, 1928) makes repeated and extended reference to witch-midwives and their iniquities; we shall return to this shortly. The eminent Jean Bodin, a sixteenth-century judge who tried many witches, reported in 1581:

> Another notorious witch living in Verignius (where her life ended last April) was a midwife who had been accused of certain acts of witchcraft but who was acquitted; later she horribly avenged the accusation by causing the destruction of uncounted men and beasts, as we have heard from the inhabitants.

Hiltprand's textbook of midwifery (1595) said that many women of this profession were witches. Two English midwives were barred from practice in 1661 and 1677, respectively, on suspicion of witchcraft; one of them was later reinstated (Hurd-Mead, 1938). Much later, in the eastern counties of England, there was a recurring tale of the midwife who reached a confinement in an impossibly short time and hinted that a broomstick was responsible (Newman and Newman, 1939). If

---

10. Joseph Addison in *The Spectator*, No. 117. See also No. 419.

a midwife had to be called at night, two women went together. Should one be obliged to make the perilous trip alone, she carried two loaves of bread so that the devil would not cause her to lose her way (Weissbart, 1905). German midwives who traveled to their patients at night in an area near Carlsbad were escorted by men with lanterns as a precaution against a meeting with a witch (Herold, 1953).

Some of the superstitions surrounding the placenta, the umbilical cord, and, as we have seen, the caul related to witchcraft. The Würzburg regulations for midwives as issued in 1555 forbade them either to carry off or to bury the placenta, and specified that it be cast into running water. Both the fanatical Martin Delrio and Guaccius in his *Compendium maleficarum* speak of the use in the Black Mass of candles made of pitch or of the umbilical cord of an infant. The Brandenburg regulations issued for midwives in 1711 specifically forbade these women to hand on or sell the fetal membranes, placenta, or umbilical cord, as these would be used in dark and nefarious manner. The *Abrégé de l'embryologie sacrée,* also dating from the eighteenth century, cites an ordinance of the Church which makes the same restriction: midwives "will never give a portion of the placenta to anyone for superstitious purposes." [11] The repetition of this prohibition certainly implies that it was not always observed, and indeed it must sometimes have been easy for the midwife, if she dared, to steal the byproducts of childbirth.

Just as witchcraft at its roots, according to Murray (1937), was essentially a pagan and debased religion—the worship of the devil—so attendance at the witches' sabbath, at which the rites of worship were performed, was a fundamental duty and privilege for the witch. Whether attendance was actual or, as sometimes (see below), no more than a drug-induced delusion, it was customary first for the devotee to smear his or her unclothed body with an unguent, the famous "witch's ointment" or "flying ointment" (Chesnel, 1856.) Grillot de Givry (1929) says that in Arras in 1460 several individuals accused of witchcraft confessed that when they were ready to attend the sabbath, they rubbed the ointment on their bodies, "then flew off where they wished, past beautiful cities, woods, and streams, and the Devil carried them to the place where they were to have their assembly." A typical account was that of Jehanette Otheniaz of Basel, as reported by Diricq

11. Cotta (1616), Delrio (1608), Dinouart (1774), Guaccius (1626), Krauss (1913), Lammert (1869).

(1910): She went to the sabbath at night, carried by the devil on his back. Sometimes he took the form of an animal; at other times she smeared a rod with an unguent supplied by the devil and was transported by this wand. She flew out of her house, she said, by either the chimney or the window. This woman died at the stake on 25 May 1597.

About 1590 Boguet (1929) quoted an earlier authority, de Lancre, to the effect that the flying ointments were either concocted by the witches or were supplied by the devil. Usually the ointments included the fat of infants. Martin Delrio, relentless pursuer of witches, asserts (1608) that at the sabbath the devil was accustomed "to smear the front of [his] staff with an ointment compounded of various strange things, chiefly the fat of slain infants." So that the supply of ointment would be plentiful, "a large number of infants are slaughtered." [12] Here speaks the fanatic. Wier (1579), ever the skeptic, nevertheless also reports a tale of the use of infant's fat in a brew. There is no doubt that such ointments were prepared and that the fat of babies was considered an essential ingredient. Since it was greatly preferred, if not imperative, that the baby not have been baptised, the body of a newborn child usually had to be procured.[13]

The composition of the flying ointment is of interest in view of its real and alleged effects. Jerome Cardan (1554), physician, mathematician, and gambler, tells how the illusions described by the witches were induced.

> Just as the [good] dinner which has been eaten makes sleep [i.e. dreaming] pleasant, so colewort [a kind of cabbage] makes it sad, pulse makes it restless, and garlic makes it dreadful. Hence from such things is born the belief of the witches, who by consuming parsley, chestnuts, beans, onions, colewort, and peas see themselves in their sleep carried to various places and there affected in

12. Sometimes witches prepared charms which were supposed to keep them from confessing under torture. At her trial in Forfar, Scotland, in September 1661, a certain Hellen Guthrie stated that she, a man, and several women "at ane of the meitings went up to the church wall about the southeist doore, and raisit a young bairn unbaptised." They made a pie of part of his body so that they "by that meins might never mack a confessione (as they thought) of their witchcraft" (Kinloch, 1848). Crossley (1845) quotes similar testimony from another case. The stealing of parts of dead infants by witches was charged by Cotta (1616) and others. The law against witchcraft passed in 1603 under James I had specified that if any person or persons "take up any dead man woman or child out of his her or theire grave, or any other place where the dead bodie resteth, or the skin bone or any other part of any dead person, to be imployed or used in any manner of Witchcraft Sorcerie Charme or Inchantment," they would commit a felony punishable by death.

13. Boguet (1929), Lea (1939), Murray (1921), Scot (1930), Summers (1928).

various ways according to the season. Therefore they take delight in this ointment, which they smear all over themselves. It consists, if it is to be believed, of the fat of infants torn from graves and the juices of parsley and nightshade, as well as of cinquefoil and soot. Incredibly they [the witches] may persuade themselves that they have seen large areas, theaters, green gardens, fishing, garments, adornments, dancing, handsome young men, and lovemaking of whatever kind they most desire.

Cardan's contemporary, Giovanni Baptista della Porta (1560), gave a comparable description of the *Lamiarum unguenta,* or witches' ointments:

> They [the witches] take the fat of infants from a watery decoction in a brazen vessel, [fat] which is left after the final boiling off and settling of the mixture, whereupon they collect and preserve it for their continuing benefit: with this they mix eleoselinum [celery], aconitum, poplar leaves, and soot. Or ANOTHER [formula] is thus: sium [a kind of parsley], common sweet flag, cinquefoil, bat's blood, deadly nightshade, and grease, and they mix these diverse ingredients. . . . So they [the witches] are seen on moonlight nights being born off through the air to banquets, sounds [of music], dancing & lovemaking of handsome young people, all the things which they most greatly desire. So great is the power of imagination, the manifestation of impressions, that that part of [their] brains which is said [to contain] memory is full of this kind of thing.

The similarity of these two passages suggests that both were drawn from a common and still earlier source. The ointment was discussed by a number of sixteenth- and seventeenth-century authorities, among them Valsalvor (Holzinger, 1883) and Francis Bacon (1676). The latter says:

> The *Oyntment* that *Witches* use, is reported to be made of the *Fat of Children* digged out of their *Graves;* of the *Juyces of Smallage* [wild celery], *Wolf-Bane* [aconite], *Cinquefoil,* mingled with the *Meal* of *Fine Wheat.* But, I suppose, that the *Soporiferous Medicines* are likest to do it; which are *Henbane* [hyoscyamus],

Hemblock, Mandrake, Moon shade [Solanum], Tobacco, Opium, Saffron, Poplar-leaves; &c.[14]

Several studies have been made of the possible pharmacological effects of the ingredients of the "flying ointments." It is debatable whether aqueous preparations of these substances would pass through the skin, but percutaneous absorption of some of the drugs when they are incorporated in a fatty or greasy base is quite possible.[15] Thus the fat was an essential component. Absorption is most effective through hairy, thin skin, and it is noteworthy that in the Arras confession, mentioned above, of persons accused of sorcery, application of the ointment was as follows. *Ils ondaient une vergue de bois bien petite, et leurs palmes et leurs mains, puis, mectoient celle verguelte entre leurs jambes* [with a small wooden wand they smeared both their hands and their palms, then placed this little wand between their legs]—that is, the ointment was applied in some of the most absorptive cutaneous sites (Grillot de Givry, 1929). Scot says that the witches "rubbe all parts of their bodys exsceedinglie, till they looke red, and be varie hot, so as the pores may be opened, and their flesh soluble and loose. They joine herewithall fat, or oile in steed thereof, that the force of the ointment maie the rather pearse inwardly, and so be more effectuall" (1886).

Soot often appeared as an ingredient, perhaps because the color seemed appropriate. It is unlikely that the bat's blood and some of the herbs had any effect, but for such plants as *Aconitum* (monkshood) and deadly nightshade it was a different story (Marzell, 1963). Aconite depresses the cardiovascular system, acts on the central nervous system, and produces sensory paralysis. It can be absorbed through the skin to give a systemic effect (Sollmann, 1957). Atropine, present in deadly nightshade and also absorbable percutaneously when in a suitable base (Clark, 1921), in sufficient doses causes excitement, delirium, and unconsciousness. Henbane and moonshade contain powerful narcotic and hallucinogenic agents. There can be little doubt that the ointments could product the illusions of the vivid experiences which the witches described, especially, as Norman points out, when

14. Schindler (1858) and Holzinger (1883) have enumerated many other plants which were used in witch ointments.
15. Clark (1921), Conklin (1958), Marzell (1963), Norman (1933), Sollmann (1957).

the ointments were used by highly suggestible and sometimes unstable individuals.[16]

Chesnel (1856) relates that in 1545 an ointment was found in the possession of a sorcerer who had been arrested. The physicians of Pope Julius III tested the substance by applying it to the body of a woman suffering from a nervouse disease. She slept for thirty-six hours, then awoke to describe various strange but pleasant hallucinations. Atropine may have been an ingredient of this ointment. Scot (1930) quotes Porta to the effect that a witch offered in prison to demonstrate the ointment, smeared herself with it, "fell down through the force of those soporiferous or sleepie ointments into a most sound and heavie sleepe," and could not be roused even by a severe beating. When she awoke, she described travels "over both seas and mountains." A Swedish couple and their dog in 1793 ate pieces of bread smeared with a black witch's ointment which had been discovered in a sawed-off cow's horn. They were observed to sleep for several hours, then to make violent movements. Later the couple reported hallucinations of flight (Gentz, 1957).

Late in the nineteenth century one experimenter failed to produce hallucinations either after rubbing himself with a fatty ointment containing aconite or taking doses of belladonna, stramonium, or atropine by mouth (Snell, 1891). However, in more recent clinical studies, dreams and hallucinations of bizarre figures, flights through the air, strange landscapes, feasts, etc. were experienced when investigators were injected with scopolamine or smeared with the ointment described by Porta, with a tincture of celery, aconite, and nightshade, or with other ingredients of the witches' ointments. On awakening, severe headaches and a sensation of fatigue were experienced (Marzell, 1963; Römpp, 1946).

Thus it is a plausible theory, suggested long ago by Reginald Scot, that if a witch wished to attend the sabbath, her ignorant mind already filled with expectations of the great event, she needed only to smear her body with one of the potent ointments known to the elect. Soon she would experience hallucinations, sink into delirium, and next day awaken exhausted by what she supposed had been her long journey.

Since there was much popular interest in witchcraft, it of course made its way into literature, and there one finds childbirth superstitions, the witch-midwife, and the witches' ointment. Rösslin, in the

16. Chesnel (1856), Marzell (1963), Norman (1933).

preface to his *Der swangern Frawe[n] und hebamme[n] rosz-garte[n]*, one of the earliest European printed works on obstetrics, devotes much of a rather long poem to the iniquities of the midwife (Klein, 1902; Rösslin, 1513). Although he does not actually call her a witch, he accuses her of destroying children "far and wide" and depriving them of holy baptism. Later in the sixteenth century John Bale wrote *A Newe Comedye or Enterlude/Concernying Thre Lawes* (1562). In the second act "Idolotria" boasts:

> And a good mydwyfe perde
> Yonge chyldren can I charme:
> With whysperynges and whychynges
> With crossynges and with kyssynges
> With blasynges and with blessynges
> That sprytes do them no harme.

Thomas Middleton drew heavily on Scot's *The Discoverie of Witchcraft* when in 1609 or 1610 he wrote his lurid play, *The Witch* (Fletcher, 1896; Middleton, 1950). In Act I, Scene 2, Hecate is directing the preparation of the brew which was a professional specialty:

> *Hec.* there take this vn-baptized-Brat
> Boile it well: preserve the ffat,
> you know 'tis pretious to transfer
> our 'noynted fflesh into the Aire,
> in Moone-light nights, or Steeple-Tops.

A little later the following ingredients for the witches' ointment were mentioned:

> I thrust in *Eleoselinum* lately
> *Aconitum, frondes populeus* and *Soote* . . .
> then *Sium, Acharum, Vulgaro* too
> *Dentaphillon,* the Blood of a fflitter-mowse
> *Solanum Somniferum et Oleum.*

The recipes apparently are directly from Porta (see above). The *oleum* of course was of human origin. A few pages farther on, Hecate's son remarks that someone "stumbled at a Pikin of Childes Greaze," and in Act V, Scene 3, she informs the audience, by this time spellbound on their benches by gruesome detail and no doubt enjoying every moment, how she feeds the ravens and screech owls which fly by her door—"I give 'em Barley, soak'd in Infants-Blood."

Shakespeare is thought to have derived many of the witchcraft details in *Macbeth* (written about 1605 but not published until 1623) from Scot's book and from records of Scottish witchcraft trials (Craig, 1932). If indifferently acted, the witches' "incantation scene" now seems rather silly. Probably this passage was not humorous to seventeenth-century playgoers. It is an interesting possibility that at more than one performance a real witch in the audience listened critically to the actor-witches on the stage as they recited the ingredients of their brew:

> Finger of birth-strangled babe
> Ditch-deliver'd by a drab.

Could ten words call up a more vivid picture?

In writing *The Lancashire Witches* (1691) Thomas Shadwell drew all technical details—and the play is crammed with them—from well-known books on witchcraft. In the preface he tells us,

> there is not one Action in the Play, nay scarce a word concerning it, but is borrow'd from some Antient, or Modern Witchmonger Which you will find in the Notes, wherein I have presented you a great part of the Doctrine of Witchcraft, believe it who will. For my part, I am (as it is said of Surly in the Alchymist) somewhat costive of belief. The Evidences I have represented are natural, viz. slight, and frivolous, such as poor old Women were wont to be hang'd upon.

Mother Demdike, a witch (and a character said to have been drawn from life), boasts (Act I):

> To a Mothers Bed I softly crept,
> And while th' unchristn'd Brat yet slept,
> I suckt the breath and bloud of that,
> And stole anothers flesh and fat
> Which I will boyl before it stink;
> The thick for Oyntment, thin for drink.

As we have seen in earlier chapters, the midwife who was not a witch sometimes resorted to spells and charms to protect and help the parturient woman and her infant. Special birth girdles were worn by the ancient Britons; Aveling (1872) believed that the rituals which accompanied application of the girdles had come from the Druids. The use of birth girdles persisted into the Christian era. A letter of inventory of the sacred relics at the convent of St. Austin in Bristow, England, in 1536 states in part:

> I send you also our Ladies girdle of Bruton, red silk. Which is a solemn relic, sent to women travailing, which shall not miscarry *in partu*. I send you also Mary Magdalene's girdle: and that is wrapped and covered with white: sent also with great reverence to women travailing. Which girdle Matilda the Empress, founder of Ferley, gave unto them, as saith the holy father of Ferley. [Strype, 1822]

In 1536 it was reported that parts of garments said to have belonged to various saints were venerated by pregnant women or used by them as aids in childbirth (Frere and Kennedy, 1910). However, both the Catholic and the Reformation Church struck out at such remnants of the superstition of earlier years. Specific attention was directed in the sixteenth century to the detection by church officials of any persons using charms at the time of childbirth, e.g.:

> Nor to use any Girdels, Purses, Mesures of our Lady, or such other Superstitious Things, to be occupied about the Woman while she laboureth, to make her beleve to have the better Spede by it (Burnet, 1715).

Scottish criminal law also forbade the use of charms for any purpose, since their effects

> cannot be produced without the Devil, and that he will not imploy himself at the desire of any who have not resigned themselves wholly to him, it is very just that the users of these should be punished, being guilty at least of Apostasie and Heresie. [Mackenzie, 1678]

In 1591 a woman named Ewfame McCalzane was brought to trial in Scotland for witchcraft even though she was the daughter of Lord Cliftounhall, a distinguished public figure. Among other offenses, she was

> Indytit, of consulting and seiking help att the said Anny Sampsoune, ane notorious Wich, for relief of your payne in the tyme of

the birth of youre twa sonnes; and ressaving [receiving] fra hir to that effect, ane boirdstane [bored stone], to be layit under the bowster [bolster], putt under your heid, Inchantit mwildis [17] and powder put in ane peice paipar, to be vsit and rowit [rolled] in your hair; and at the tyme of your drowis [birth pangs], your guidmannis sark [husband's shirt] to be presentlie tane of him, and laid woumplit [folded up] under your bedseit. The quhilk [which] being praktesit be yow, as ye had ressavit the samin fra [received the same from] the said Annie, and the information of the vse thairof; your seiknes wes cassin of you [your sickness was cast from you], unnaturallie, in the birth of youre fyrst sone, vpoune ane dog [upon a dog]; quhilk ranne away and wes newir sene agane: And in the birth of your last sone, the same prakteis foirsaid wes vsit, and your naturall and kindlie payne unnaturallie cassin of yow, vpoun the wantoune catt in the hous; quhilk lyke wyis, wes newir sene thaireftir.

In other words, it was charged that by the use of charms the pains of childbirth were transferred from Ewfame McCalzane in one instance into a dog and in another into a cat. The unfortunate woman was convicted on this and other charges and died at the stake (Dalyell, 1834; Pitcairn, 1833).

Because midwives so often were in bad repute, even an innocent practitioner might be accused of witchcraft if the delivery had an unhappy outcome or if the nonobstetrical patients whom some midwives attempted to treat did not recover. For example, a certain Ursley Kemp, midwife, nurse, and remover of spells from the sick, was brought to court as a witch in 1582 apparently just because she was a suspicious character (Notestein, 1911). One of the depositions in the records at York Castle reads

CXXIV. Mrs. Pepper. For Using Charms, Etc. Feb. 3, 1664–5, Newcastle-on-Tyne, before Sir Francis Liddle, Kt., mayor. Margaret, *wife of Robert Pyle, pittman,* sayeth, that aboute halfe a yeare

17. "Inchantit mwildis" was "powder maid of mens joyntis and memberis, in Natoun Kirk," it was alleged in the indictment against Agnes Sampson, who was also executed for witchcraft. A famous midwife, "the wise wife of Keith," near Edinburgh, she was said to be intelligent and "matron like, grave and settled in her answers, which were all to some purpose" (Dalyell, 1834). She was charged with supplying the pain-removing powder both to Ewfame McCalzane and to a Lady Hirmestoune "the nycht of the delyverie of hir birth" (Pitcairn, 1833).

agoe, her husband, being not well, sent his water to Mrs. Pepper, a midwife, and one that uses to cast water.

That is, Mrs. Pepper professed to diagnose illness by examination of the patient's urine. She was charged with having bewitched Pyle but seems to have been found not guilty.

The devil, according to the Augsburg *Hebammenordnung,* could trick the midwife into using incantations. A priest in Breslau no doubt summed up popular opinion in 1494: *in partu obstetrices mille demonica operantur similiter et partientes* (in childbirth the midwives are busy with a thousand devilish things as well as with the women in travail) (Bächtold-Stäubli, 1931).

Even more serious were the charges that midwives destroyed infants before or just after birth (Thompson, 1929). Such accusations were recorded as early as about 1460 (Lea, 1939). Part I, Question XI, of the *Malleus maleficarum* charges that witch-midwives destroy the child *in utero,* causing an abortion, or find a moment of privacy in which to offer the newborn infant to Satan. In Strasburg, the book relates, a mother who refused the services of a certain midwife was subsequently bewitched and suffered greatly. A Swiss midwife was said to have confessed the murder of over forty infants by piercing their heads with a needle during delivery. Again and again the authors of the *Malleus maleficarum* accuse witch-midwives of infanticide and refer to them in condemnatory terms—"commit most horrid crimes . . . surpass all other witches in their crimes" (Summers, 1928). It is difficult, even impossible, to separate the actual from the imagined offenses, but there can be no doubt of the utter vindictiveness toward any midwife who was suspect.

The charge that witch-midwives killed fetuses and newborn infants was repeated by others (Chereau, 1881). What made the crime even blacker was the delusion that Satan thus was able to steal the soul of the unbaptized baby (Murray, 1918). Frommann's *Tractatus de fascinatione* (1575) says, "The Devil arranges through the midwives not only the abortive death of the fetuses lest they be brought to the holy font of baptism, but also by their [the midwives'] aid he causes newborn babies secretly to be consecrated to himself."[18] Lea (1939)

18. If it was discovered that an infant had been promised to the devil, a benevolent midwife could break the charm on the sixth night after birth by placing a holy candle inside a circle drawn on the floor, cutting a lock of hair from the baby, and throwing the hair to the Evil One (Bächtold-Stäubli, 1931).

quotes from Jaquier's *Flagellum hereticorum fascinariorum* of 1581 a charge that midwives often strangle the newborn child on command of the Evil One, one woman thus having, she confessed, prevented the baptism of twenty-three babies. Three of the women tried for witch-craft at Schongau, Bavaria, in 1589 were midwives; one of them is said to have stated that she could cause the death of the fetus *in utero* (Höfler, 1893). Boguet (1929) makes a similar charge and adds that the midwife may offer the newborn child to Satan and then kill it by thrusting a bodkin into the brain. The accusation appears again in Hiltprandum's book on midwifery (1595) and in Guaccius' *Compendium maleficarum* of 1626. The latter continues:

> Moreover, when they do not kill the babies, they offer them (horrible to relate) to the demons in this execrable manner. After the child is born the witch-midwife, if the lying-in mother is not alone, pretends that something should be done to restore the strength of the baby, carries it outside the bedroom, and elevating it on high, [offers] it to the Prince of Devils, that is to say, Lucifer, and to all the others.

Such a consecration to the Evil One was also reported to have occurred in Scotland. The justices of the peace, it was said, were observed in conversation with the devil; one of the justices was alleged to have handed over his newborn only child, "stepping out with it in his arms to the staircase, where the devil stood ready, as it was suspected, to receive the innocent victim" (Sharpe, 1884).

Closely related to the idea that the soul of the unbaptized baby could be lost to the devil was the belief that it was a fairy's trick to steal a newborn, unbaptized infant, perhaps leaving a "changeling," a soulless and misshapen child of the fairies, in the human baby's place (Hastings, 1910).[19] Infants with congenital defects were sometimes believed to be changelings. Some inhabitants of Scotland believed that every seven years the fairies had to pay "the teind to hell," a tribute to the devil of a fairy baby, unless the fairies could steal and substitute a human infant (Gregor, 1881). Shakespeare and Spenser allude to changelings.[20]

19. There are also many folktales about human midwives who deliver fairy babies (Hartland, 1890), but the substitution of changelings seems not to be a feature of such stories. Midwives who assisted fairies in labor were handsomely rewarded, but failure to cooperate often meant death by drowning (Weissbart, 1905).

20. *Midsummer Night's Dream*, II.1.20 and 120; *Winter's Tale*, III.3.122. *Faerie Queene*, I.10.65 (Thiselton Dyer, 1883).

The greatest dread of those who waited by the woman in travail was that she and her child might lose their souls (Hull, 1928). As Hastings (1910) remarks, "the mother is no longer a real Christian until she is churched, for she has been despoiled of her Christianity by the child in the act of birth." The child was not a Christian until it was properly baptized. Until this protection was conferred, the infant was considered to be in deadly peril from the powers of evil. Further, Margaret Murray points out, there is clear proof that "the personage called by Christian writers 'the Devil,' was considered by the witches themselves to be God incarnate as a man. To this deity they made sacrifices of various kinds, the most important of such sacrifices being that of a child." It was essential that the child be unbaptized and therefore still outside the Christian church (Murray, 1918). This, according to the writings of Scot and Boguet, was why the witches and witch-midwives made every effort to obtain the infant before baptism, although Scot did reject Bodin's notion that "witches sacrifice their own children to the devil before baptism."[21] Wier (1564) quotes another authority to the effect that the witches "lie in wait for infants not yet baptized, or actually baptized, particularly when they are not protected by the sign of the cross and prayers"—that is, when they have been improperly baptized. Thus supernatural dangers surrounded the unborn infant, the unbaptized baby, and the "unchurched" mother and, as a result, hosts of protective practices and devices were developed.[22] Fear of the Evil One of course provided an urgent reason for prompt baptism. The other reason was the traditional belief that at best the soul of an unbaptized child must abide forever in limbo.

When others could not help, it became an obligation of the midwife to see that the baby was properly baptized. If a priest was not at hand and it was evident that the newborn infant would not long survive, someone, the midwife if necessary, was expected to take the baby to the priest. The renowned midwife Mme. Le Boursier de Coudray in her manual, *Abrégé de l'art des accouchements* (1777), remarks ruefully: "There is usually some danger in carrying infants to baptism during the night, especially in the rural parishes: the bad roads, ditches, planks, places one must jump over, ice, bad weather, encounters with dogs &c." In an emergency, properly qualified midwives were authorized and in-

---

21. Boguet (1929), Scot (1930). It is probable that Scot himself did not believe in witches and that he was simply quoting the opinions of others.
22. Hastings (1910), Henderson (1879), Martin (1934), Sébillot (1906).

structed to baptize the baby according to the laws of the Church,[23] as they may to this day. In the British Museum Library is a very rare and fragile pamphlet, dating from about 1530, entitled *Eyn unterricht für die hebammen / wie sie in der not Tauffen sollen* (Instructions for midwives as to how they should baptize in case of need) (Anon.). Rösslin, the sixteenth-century obstetrician, held the midwife responsible if the baby died without proper baptism and was consequently never admitted to salvation (Klein, 1902; Rösslin, 1513).

An interesting case is recorded in the Consistorial Acts of the diocese of Rochester, England:

> 1523, Oct. 14—Eliz. Gaynsford, *obstetrix, examinat' dicit in vim juramenti sui sub hac forma verborum* [midwife, being examined, testified under oath as follows].—"I, the aforesaid Elizabeth, seeing the child of Tho. Everey, late born in jeopardy of life, by the authorite of my office, then beyng midwyfe, dyd christen the same childe under this manner, In the name of the Fader, the Son, and the Holy Ghost, I christen thee Denys, *issundend' meram aquam super caput infantul.*"—*Interrogata erat,*[24] whether the child was born and delivered from the wyfe of the said Thomas; whereto she answereth and saith, that the childe was not born for she saw nothyng of the childe but the hedde, and for perell the childe was in, and in that tyme of nede, she christened as is aforesaid, and cast water on the childe's hede. After which so done the child was born, and was had to the churche, where the Priest gave to it that chrystynden that takkyd, and the childe is yet alyf.

An East Sussex parish register: "1579. Was baptized Joan Birmingham, the daughter of John Birmingham and Joan his wife, by the midwife at home, and it was buried on the 20th day." Another: "St. Mary's Litchfield, Oct. 12, 1591. Margarett, dr. of Walter Henningham de Pypehall, baptized by the midwife, and, as yet not broughte to ye churche to be there examined and testified by them that were present."[25]

It is interesting that baptism by the midwife in case of urgent necessity had the sanction of the Church as early as the seventh century.

23. Barnes (1903), Blencowe (1851), Burn (1797, 1829), Burnet (1865), Dinouart (1774), Ferraris (1746), Gasparri (1933), van Espen (1784).

24. Correcting the first word as copied and without the contractions, the Latin would read *effundendam meracam aquam super caput infantuli:—Interrogata erat* (Pouring pure water on the head of the infant:—she was asked).

25. Aveling (1872), Blencowe (1851), W. and D. (1785).

Aveling quotes a ruling in the *Liber poenitentialis* of Theodore, Archbishop of Canterbury: *Mulier baptizare non praesumat, nisi cogenti necessitate maxima* (The woman may not presume to baptize except when compelled by extreme necessity). A decree of the Council of Bourges in 1584 (Titre IX, Can. 8) is similar: "Neither midwives nor lay persons may anticipate baptism, nor may they presume to confer it, except in extreme necessity and evident danger." The midwife was bound under peril of mortal sin to know and to use the proper ritual when she baptized an infant, and the clergy was specifically charged with instruction of midwives in the administration of this rite. Baptisms, it is said, were performed by some English midwives until early in the seventeenth century, although it appears that by 1577 the practice had been forbidden in Protestant households.[26]

Both church and state made strenuous efforts to regulate the practice of midwifery. The first municipal ordinances for this purpose are believed to be those in the *Hebammenordnung* of Regensburg, Germany, dating from 1452.[27] The earliest German ecclesiastical regulations recorded appear to be the Würzburg Synodal Statutes of 1491 (Bächtold-Stäubli, 1931), although the *Malleus maleficarum* had earlier directed (Part III, Question 34) that magistrates should permit only good Catholics to serve as midwives (Summers, 1928).

In general the ordinances dealt with the proper training of the midwife, her equal availability to rich and poor, the circumstances in which she should seek the help of a physician, and other professional questions. But regularly evident was a continuing concern lest she indulge in "superstitious methods" or outright witchcraft. Under the Würzburg statutes, "the midwife hereby is strictly prohibited from employment of any superstitious practices." Würtemburg in 1552 forbade "superstitious sayings or other ungodliness" during the delivery. Regensburg specified that any "midwife who employs magic or superstitious methods shall accordingly be beaten on her body." The *Gothäische Landesordnung* of 1658 prohibited witchcraft at childbirth. The *Würzburg–Mainz–Wormser Kirchenordnung* of 1670 specified that "no one is permitted either to induce or to palliate the birth or to employ superstitious methods for mother or child." Similar wording appears in a German ordinance of the eighteenth century. The frequent reference by

26. Aveling (1872), Balard (1924), Burnet (1715), Delaunay (1921), Dinouart (1774), Ferraris (1746), Frere and Kennedy (1910), Raine (1850).
27. Burckhard (1912), Ditton (1930), Höfler (1893).

the regulations to witchcraft leaves little doubt that the midwives continued to fall under suspicion.[28] Church law added the requirement that "Those baptized by the midwives are to be re-baptized in instances when the midwives are suspected of witchcraft." In addition, German midwives were obliged to take oaths of office in which they swore to avoid superstitious practices.[29]

French authorities likewise recognized the need for close supervision of the midwives, and specified that they receive professional and religious instruction and take an oath. In the smaller communities the midwife was sometimes selected by the priest from among the virtuous older women of the parish; requirements were that she "had never been suspected of heresy or witchcraft," or that she be "free of all suspicion of heresy, witchcraft, superstition, or any other crime whatsoever, and finally that she be of exemplary life and morals." The methods for selection of the midwife and for her subsequent instruction in the form of baptism were specified by ecclesiastical regulations.[30]

The regulation of midwives began somewhat later in Britain than in Germany and will be recounted in a later chapter.

All the evidence considered, what can we conclude? It is well established that witchcraft was widely practiced in Europe, and we can be sure that some midwives were tempted to enjoy its forbidden delights. Undoubtedly there were opportunities for them to use witchcraft professionally. They were often accused of practicing the black arts, sometimes unjustly but sometimes, it appears, quite correctly. What proportion of the midwives was involved in witchcraft cannot be determined. The records, even when factual, are chiefly accounts of wrongdoing. Then as now, good deeds went unnumbered, and we must presume that law-abiding midwives, if not unrewarded, still were usually not mentioned. Probably the considerable majority abided conscientiously by the regulations. Perhaps the most convincing evidence that some did not, is indirect—the manifest concern of both local governments and the Church, which for more than three hundred years by municipal ordinance, episcopal injunction, pastoral exhortation, examination, and oath sought to stay the midwife from "all manner of witchcraft, charm or sorcery."

28. As late as 1814 the municipal ordinances of Basel, Switzerland, forbade midwives to use superstitious methods.

29. Anon. (1739), Bächtold-Stäubli (1931), Burckhard (1911, 1912), Ferraris (1746), Kern (1929). Long before, Soranus had warned about the superstitious midwife (Temkin, 1956).

30. Balard (1924), Delaunay (1921), Gosset (1909).

Perrette
the Midwife

Most of the accounts of midwives charged with witchcraft are records of their trials, and most of the trials ended in the death sentence. This true story is a happy exception. The original record is set down in the stiff legal phrases and interminable sentences of a contemporary document of the Court of France.[1] A literal translation does not tell all that happened, except by implication, and the following account, although based entirely on the record, is therefore in my own words.

At the beginning of the fifteenth century there lived in Paris a midwife named Perrette. She and her husband, Thomas of Rouen, had had fifteen children. What was more remarkable for that day was that all the children were still alive. So Perrette worked hard at her profession to support herself, her children, and her elderly husband who, apparently, was not successful in his trade as a minstrel. Perrette had taken her oath as midwife and followed her profession in Paris for over twenty years. Unlike some of her colleagues, she had made a fine reputation, and had a devoted clientele among women of her own class as well as the nobility. In the days when wives expected to bear many

1. In the Wellcome Medical Historical Library in London I came by good fortune on the *Biographie des sages-femmes célèbres, anciennes, modernes et contemporaines,* by A. Delacoux, Docteur en Médecine de la Faculté de Paris, etc., published in Paris by Trinquart and Delacoux in 1834. On pp. 130–37 appear a portrait and the account of Perrette. Most of the Delacoux account is repeated by Witkowski (1891), but neither book is now readily accessible. Perrette's story is told originally in her letter of pardon, which Delacoux found in "the registry of charters in the historical section of the Royal Archives," presumably in Paris. The document is number 223; its title is *Remissio pro Perreta uxore Thome de Rothomago.* Delacoux quotes the letter in extenso.

children, an expert and reliable midwife was a useful person to count among one's friends. The time was coming when Perrette's good name and the devotion of her patrons were to meet a desperate need.

On day late in June 1407 a woman named Jehanne Chantre came to see Perrette. They were well acquainted, for Jehanne, nicknamed *La Boudière*,[2] had delivered three of Perrette's children; evidently Perrette had confidence in her. La Boudière had an attractive but highly illegal and dangerous proposition: she would, she promised, pay twenty crowns for the body of a stillborn infant. Why she did not herself procure the body and keep this handsome sum is not explained. Perhaps she was no longer in practice, or perhaps she was afraid. At any rate, Perrette refused in horror, as well she might; the request smacked of one of those acts of witchcraft which, she well knew, could mean a horrible exit from this world and damnation in the next. Also, added Perrette, she did not know where to obtain the body.

But Jehanne was persistent, and after a while revealed the rest of the story. In Paris there was a great lord who had recently been forced to terminate his attendance at Court because he had discovered he had leprosy. Facing not only a frightening disease but rejection from all society, he was desperate. Then he had found a quack physician who promised a cure—but the cure required the body of an infant. So the twenty shining crowns were offered, with the further promise that if the nobleman did recover he would pay Perrette so handsomely that she would never again have to leave home, on a busy day or a rainy night, to deliver another baby. Even if she had doubts about this last, the prospect of twenty crowns, ten times what she earned at a confinement, joined with the urging of her friend and frantic requests from the leprous lord, overcame her better judgment, and she consented.

But procuring the body seemed to be impossible. Time passed. Jehanne came almost daily to Perrette's house, urging speed. In desperation Perrette disclosed the secret to a third midwife, Katherine, known to her friends as *La Petionne*.[3] Perrette thought that perhaps Katherine could supply the body, but discovered that Jehanne had already approached La Petionne without success. Still Jehanne kept returning to Perrette. Tempers grew short, and finally, late in August Perrette snapped out that she could not obtain the body, had no idea how to get one, and washed her hands of the whole sorry affair.

2. Slang for "midwife."
3. Slang for "the little one."

This dangerous episode might have ended there. But the nobleman was still sick, and the image of the twenty glittering coins would not fade. One day about six weeks after Perrette withdrew from her agreement, she was visited by Katherine. When they were alone, Katherine drew from her pocket the body of a fetus no longer than a hand. "Keep this until La Boudière comes for it," she instructed, then left. Why Katherine did not deliver the tiny remains directly to Jehanne instead of involving Perrette, thus reducing Katherine's fee accordingly, is not clear. Very likely she was frightened and hoped to screen herself behind an intermediary. In any case, word soon reached Jehanne. She came to Perrette and asked if Katherine had brought the body. In answer, Perrette brought out the sad little figure. Very well, said Jehanne, she would speak to her contacts. Cannily, she left the incriminating remains with the obliging and gullible Perrette.

The secret apparently was well kept, and Perrette was not visited that night by the authorities, although she must have worried. Next day there returned not Jehanne but Katherine with the surprising remark that she did not know what the nobleman and the doctor wanted to do with the body. Pretty clearly, Katherine was by now badly frightened; she advised that they bury the body instead of delivering it. Perrette, who must have been relieved, agreed that this was a good idea, and the two women set off. They found a field, buried the body, and returned to their homes. Poor Perrette! About the time that she must have been congratulating herself on being well out of the affair, there was a knock at the door. There stood La Boudière, asking for the baby.

When she heard what Katherine and Perrette had done, Jehanne was furious. She raged at Perrette, demanding to know why the agreement had been broken and threatening that Perrette would live to be sorry. It must have been an ugly scene. Then La Boudière became more calm and begged Perrette to go with her and make excuses to those who wished to buy the body.

Once more Perrette, "who is a simple woman," gave in. She was apparently one of those compliant people who never learn to refuse. In spite of the abuse, she went obligingly with Jehanne to an inn in the rue de Rosiers where they met with three strangers, "a tall nobleman dressed in gray, and another less important gentleman also dressed in gray, and another dressed in black." When Jehanne explained that Perrette and Katherine had indeed had a body but had buried it, the three men were enraged. Perrette was threatened with exposure and physical injury. Then the nobleman in gray (Perrette later heard him spoken to as Guiselin de Rebesnes) changed his approach and begged her to help him. He swore solemnly that the baby was not wanted for any evil purpose but only to provide a little ointment for the sores on the face of the leper. When it was all over the baby would be returned to Perrette for burial.

Again Perrette surrendered to pressure. She and a young varlet from the inn left to find the field. La Boudière, too clever to risk being caught with the body, stayed with the men. The fetus was dug up, brought back to the inn, and turned over to the man in black. He was, someone said, a doctor. Guiselin and his friend in gray looked on while La Boudière went to another room of the inn and came back with a dressing gown lined with fur. This she handed to Perrette, saying it was security for payment of her fee. Perrette trudged home with the gown, and two or three days later La Boudière turned up and exchanged the gown, not for twenty crowns but for two francs.

The record makes no comment here, but it seems clear that Jehanne was playing a very crooked game. She had avoided making direct payment to Perrette in front of the others by using the gown as security. Then later she handed over only a miserable two francs, doubtless pocketing the difference. Perrette at this point could do nothing except, perhaps, to confide in her husband, from whom the entire affair had thus far been concealed.

Even then the matter might have ended safely if the ultimate disaster had not occurred: someone told the Provost's men that the body of a stillborn infant was being used to work witchcraft, and very soon Perrette, Katherine, Guiselin, "and several others"[4] found themselves in a Paris prison. There they stayed for six weeks in what even the authorities conceded was "great privation and misery." Then they came to trial before the Provost of Paris. Perrette and Katherine escaped with their lives and without much further imprisonment,[5] but the sentence was bad enough. Both women were condemned to be "turned" on the pillory and to be deprived of the office of midwife. Two kinds of pillory were in use at this time. One was like the stocks familiar in Great Britain and later in Colonial America. The other also consisted of an apparatus for confining the neck and arms of the prisoner, but the framework was mounted on a wheel on a vertical axis. The victim

4. The document says nothing further about the infamous Boudière.
5. In 1407 the witchcraft hysteria had not yet reached full force. In later years many victims of perverted justice were executed on the basis of suspicion alone.

could thus be rotated and seen by all. The pillory of course was in a public place, and the victim was often the defenseless target of jeers, insults, and filth from the street. Katherine and Perrette endured their humiliation, and then—it must have been some time in November—they were discharged from prison. Perrette at last was free to go home, but to what? Her children were hungry. Thomas was old and had little work. Perrette was barred from her profession. Even the dry legal record shows pity—"she and her said husband had the prospect of spending the rest of their lives in reproach and dishonor and in the greatest poverty and wretchedness." Although winter was at hand and they had always lived in Paris, Thomas said that they must flee.

But now it appears that friends came to the help of the desperate family. Who the friends were, we do not know, but the record gives a hint.

> Her service, office, or skill are very necessary to the public welfare, and likewise several pregnant women place great reliance in her knowledge and diligence and from day to day come to her and ask her to deliver their children.

We can guess that the husbands of these women listened when their spouses insisted that they would have only Perrette, properly licensed or not, when the baby was due. There was but one solution. Someone, probably an educated husband, helped Perrette prepare a royal petition for pardon and reinstatement. Someone, quite possibly a noble husband, used his influence at court.

There were months of waiting and discouragement for Thomas and Perrette. Then on a day in the spring came glorious news.

> We have considered these things and wish to be merciful in this case rather than to exercise a rigorous justice. The said Perrette has always been an honest woman, leading a good life, reputable, and virtuous in speech without exception, having never been accused or suspected of making accusation or reproach. She had done or committed the above mentioned things more through simplicity and ignorance than through malice, expecting in addition that what was done would harm no one save only the law. The said Perrette, not only by her long detention in prison but also by the chastisement and disgrace of the said pillory, has been, and is, greatly punished. . . .

Therefore we have by our special grace and royal authority discharged, forgiven, and pardoned Perrette of Rouen in respect to the above mentioned case. Be it known by these presents that we do discharge, forgive, and pardon the deed, case, and offense above described, together with the deprivation of her said office, and we restore to her her good name and reputation in the said office or profession of midwife, without being sworn,[6] and her goods which were not confiscated, satisfaction to be made under civil law if any were so [confiscated]. Given by order to our Provost of Paris and to all other officials and officers or to their lieutenants present and to come, and to each one of them as it may pertain to him, that by our mercy, remission, pardon, and vindication they permit, suffer, and allow the said Perrette to live justly and peacefully, without causing her, or suffering her to be caused, sent, or given hereafter any obstacle or impediment whatsoever in body, in goods, or in the exercise of her said profession or office.[7] . . . Given at Paris the seventeenth day of May in the year of grace 1408 and of our reign the twenty-eighth.

By the King in Council. CHARRON.

6. That is, without again taking the midwife's oath of office (see next chapter).
7. Perrette lived until her death in 1411 in the rue Aubribouché, or Aubrey-le-Boucher. She was buried in the vault of her parish church, Saint-Jacques-de-la-Boucherie.

Early Regulation
of English Midwives

In spite of the importance in past centuries of the services of the midwife, regulatory measures intended to ensure for her a reasonable level of skill and professional ethics came belatedly to western Europe. In England, basic regulation of midwives evolved in the sixteenth and seventeenth centuries. Initially, the various bodies which undertook to control the practice of the midwife seem to have concerned themselves more with her character than with her ability. Both concerns were justified. We have seen how some midwives became involved in witchcraft. There were other flaws. Richard Jonas (Rösslin, 1540) remarks:

> for as touchynge mydwyfes / as there be many of them ryght expert / diligēt / wyse / circumspecte / and tender aboute suche busynesse: so be there agayne manye mo [more] full undyscreate / unreasonable / chorleshe / farre to seke in suche thynges / the whiche sholde chieflye helpe and socoure the good women in theyr most paynefull labor and thronges [distress]. Throughe whose rudenesse [and] rasshenesse onely I doubte not / but that a greate nomber are caste awaye and destroyed (the more petye).

Some provision had been available for lying-in women in fifteenth-century hospitals and monasteries, but this appears virtually to have ended with the dissolution of the religious houses under the Reformation. Deliveries occurred in private homes. Medical men seldom attended. The professional standards of the midwives were often deplorable and, indeed, sometimes could scarcely be said to exist (Garrison, 1929; Peachey, 1924). Andrew Boorde, a physician, commented in 1547 that uterine prolapse can be due to improper care in childbirth. He added that if the prolapse "do come of evyl orderynge af a woman whan that she is delivered, it muste come of an unexpert midwife." If the latter could be properly instructed, he says, "there shulde not be halfe so many women myscary, nor so many children perished in every

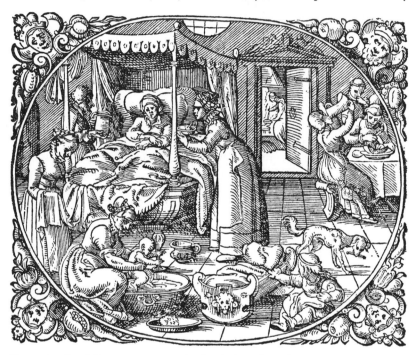

Fig. 7. Another delivery room scene, the frontispiece of Rueff's *De conceptu*. The new-born baby is bathed, food and drink are served to the mother, and the rest of the family celebrates at the dinner table.

place in Englaunde as there be." Willughby explained in 1670 that he had written his *Observations in Midwifery* in English because

> few of our midwives bee learned in severall languages. For I have been with some, that could not read; with severall, that could not write; with many, that understood very little of practice, & for such as these bee, it would no do good to speak to them of anatomizing of the womb, or to tell them of the learned workes of Mercatus, or Senertus, or Spigelius.

Elizabeth Cellier (or Celleor), a remarkable member of the profession who was not only literate but outspoken, stated in a royal petition in 1687:

> That within the space of twenty years last past, above six-thousand women have died in childbed, more than thirteen-thousand children have been abortive and about five-thousand *chrysome* infants [those in their first month of life] have been buried within the weekly bills of mortality; above two-thirds of which, amounting to sixteen thousand souls, have in all probability perished, for want of due skill and care, in those women who practice the art of midwifery. [Oldys, 1809]

The appalling maternal and infant mortality in Tudor England was, Copeman (1960) believes, a major factor in preventing a population increase at a time when the birth rate was high.

The laws of Britain, as we have seen, provided severe penalties for persons convicted of witchcraft. However, *The Statutes of the Realm* from the time of Magna Carta to the end of the reign of Queen Anne in 1714 do not mention midwives in this or any other connection (Anon., 1817, 1840).

The Church was concerned about the practice of midwifery. No doubt the failure of the state to regulate this profession was one reason for ecclesiastical concern; humanitarian considerations were not overlooked, but the overriding issue seems at first to have been the proper baptism of the infant. Should it appear that the baby might die before the priest could perform the baptism, the midwife was obliged to conduct the rite, and it was of course essential that she do so correctly (Hardouin, 1714); the midwife's obligation in this matter was explicit in ecclesiastical law.

Bishop Rowland Lee's *Injunction for Coventry and Lichfield,* dated about 1537, said that "the midwife may use it [baptism] in time of necessity; commanding the women when the time of birth draweth near, to have at all seasons a vessel of clean water for the same purpose" (Frere and Kennedy, 1910). Other clerics of the period gave similar instructions. Entries in parish registers record these baptisms.

> 1547 Ther was baptised by the Midwyffe and so buryed, the childe of Thoms. Goldhm., called Creature.[1]

1. Burn (1829) suggests that this may have been a baptism before birth.

1567, William Lawson, an infant, christend by the woemen, buryed 21 Martii [March].

The Reformation brought at least one edict, in 1577, "that no midwifes, nor any other women, be suffred to minister babtisme," but the practice continued.

> 1579. Was baptised Joan Birmingham, daughter of John Birmingham and Joan his wife, by the midwife at home, and it was buried on the 20th day.

> The seventh day of August was buryed Jone Newman, the daught. of Robert Newman, domi baptizata erat p. obstetricem [she was baptized at home by the midwife], 1583.

> Oct. 12, 1591, Margarett, D^r of Walter Henningham, de Pypehall, baptized by the mydwyfe, and as yett not broughte to ye Churche to be there examyned and testified by them that were there present.[2]

Blencowe (1851) states that for many years after the Reformation the interval between birth and baptism was very seldom more than two days.

One midwife, perhaps under stress, made on embarrassing mistake. The parish register of Hanwell, Middlesex, records:

> Thomas, son of Thomas Messenger and Elizabeth his wife, was born and baptized Oct: 24, 1731, by the midwife at the Font, called a boy, and named by the godfather, *Thomas,* but proved a girl!! [Burn, 1829]

Evidence for baptism by the midwife goes back to 1303, when Robert Mannyng of Brunne wrote, "For every man bothe hyghe and loghe / The poyntes of bapteme owet to knowe." He detailed the correct procedure, then added that midwives must understand it thoroughly. There followed the tale of a midwife who "loste a chylde both soule and lyfe" because she used the wrong words. When the priest discovered her error, "She was commaundede she shulde no more / Come eftesones where chyldryn were bore" (Mannyng, 1862), an early case of clerical regulation of midwifery.

Similar admonitions were included by John Myrc, an English canon, about 1450 in his *Instructions for Parish Priests* (1868 ed.). In specify-

2. Blencowe (1851), Burn (1797, 1829), Frere and Kennedy (1910), Raine (1850).

ing the midwife's duties in an obstetrical emergency, he lays down, possibly for the first time in England, some definite rules of professional conduct and the indications for Caesarean section:

> And teche the mydewyf neuer the latere
> That heo have redy clene watere,
> Then bydde hyre spare for no schame,
> to folowe [baptize] the chylde there at hame,
> And thaghe the chylde bote half be bore,
> Hed and necke and no more,
> Bydde hyre spare neuer the later
> to crystene hyt and caste on water;
> And but scho mowe se the hed,
> Loke scho folowe [baptize] hyt for no red;
> And ef the wommon thenne dye
> Teche the mydwyf that scho hye [hasten]
> For to vndo hyre wyth a knyf
> And for to save the chyldes lyf.
> And hye that hyt crystened be,
> For that ys a dede of charyte.

In 1512, under Henry VIII, an act was passed which permitted representatives of the Church to grant licenses for the practice of medicine and surgery to persons who had first been examined by the Bishop of London or the Dean of St. Paul's. Ecclesiastical licensing of qualified midwives probably began soon afterward. It continued until 1642. According to Elizabeth Cellier, Bishop Bonner (1500?–69?) issued the first midwife's license.[3] Andrew Boorde suggested in 1547,

> In my tyme . . . every midwife shuld be presented with honest women of great gravitie to the Byshoppe, and that they shulde testify for her that they do present shoulde be a sadde woman wise and discrete, havynge experience, and worthy to have ye office of a midwife. Than the Byshoppe with ye counsell of a doctor of phisicke ought to examin her, and to instruct her in that thinge that she is ignoraunt, and thus proved amitted [admission] is a laudable thing, for and this were used in England there shulde nat be halfe so many women myscary, nor so many children perished

3. Anon. (1895), Barnes (1903), Celleor (1687), Hurd-Mead (1938), Peachey (1900), Penny (1900), Williams (1901).

in euery place in Englaunde as there be. The byshoppes ought to loke on this matter.

Several steps were necessary before the midwife's license was issued. First, it was expected that she had acquired at least a degree of professional competence and had received proper instruction in the form of baptism. She then underwent examination by midwives and surgeons concerning her character and skill (Anon., 1895). Before one Eleonor Pead, for example, was licensed on 26 August 1567, she was questioned by Matthew, Archbishop of Canterbury, about her knowledge of mid-

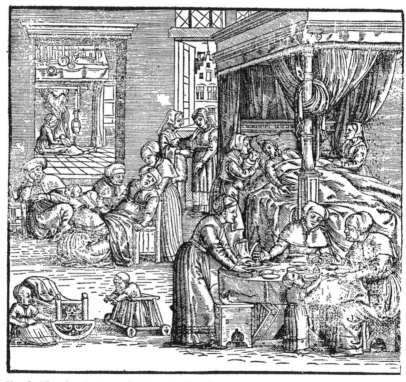

Fig. 8. The frontispiece of Walter Ryff's *Frawen Rosengarten* (Frankfurt, 1545). A woman in labor sits on the birth stool, assisted by the midwife. The delivery over, the baby is brought to the mother as she rests in a bed; the curtains are tucked back so that we can see. A meal is enjoyed by some of the attendants, and beside a cradle a small child exercises in a "walker" much like its modern counterpart. The well-populated scene includes thirteen women, a newborn infant, four small children—and no men.

ε§ Plate 1. Midwife's license. "These are to Certify those whom it may concerne that Elizabeth Davis wife of Thomas Davis of the parish of St. Catherine Creechurch in London midwife is a woman that wee knowe very well to be of a good & honest life and Conversation [behavior], & very knowing skillfull and expert in the practice of Midwifery wch office or ffunction of a midwife she has pformed for the space of eighteen yeares wth great care and good success, and in testimony hereof we have subscribed our Names." The license is signed by a minister, two churchwardens, and two midwives. At the bottom is the notation in Latin, "The witnesses and midwife took the oath 10 January 1661 in my presence"—but the surrogate neglected to add his name.

᠊᠊᠊§ Plate 2. Midwife's license. "These are to certifie that Margaret Corney widdow by practise a Midwife is a person Loyale to his Matie [Majestie] a Dutiful & obedient Daughter of ye church of England, her Mother, of knowne & experienced ability in her pfession of Midwifery as by sufficient testimony of many persons she hath delivered will be made good, & hath been an Inhabitant in this parish of St. Peter Paul's Wharf forty years." John Williams signed this as rector and again (at bottom) as surrogate. Note the ages of the two midwife witnesses.

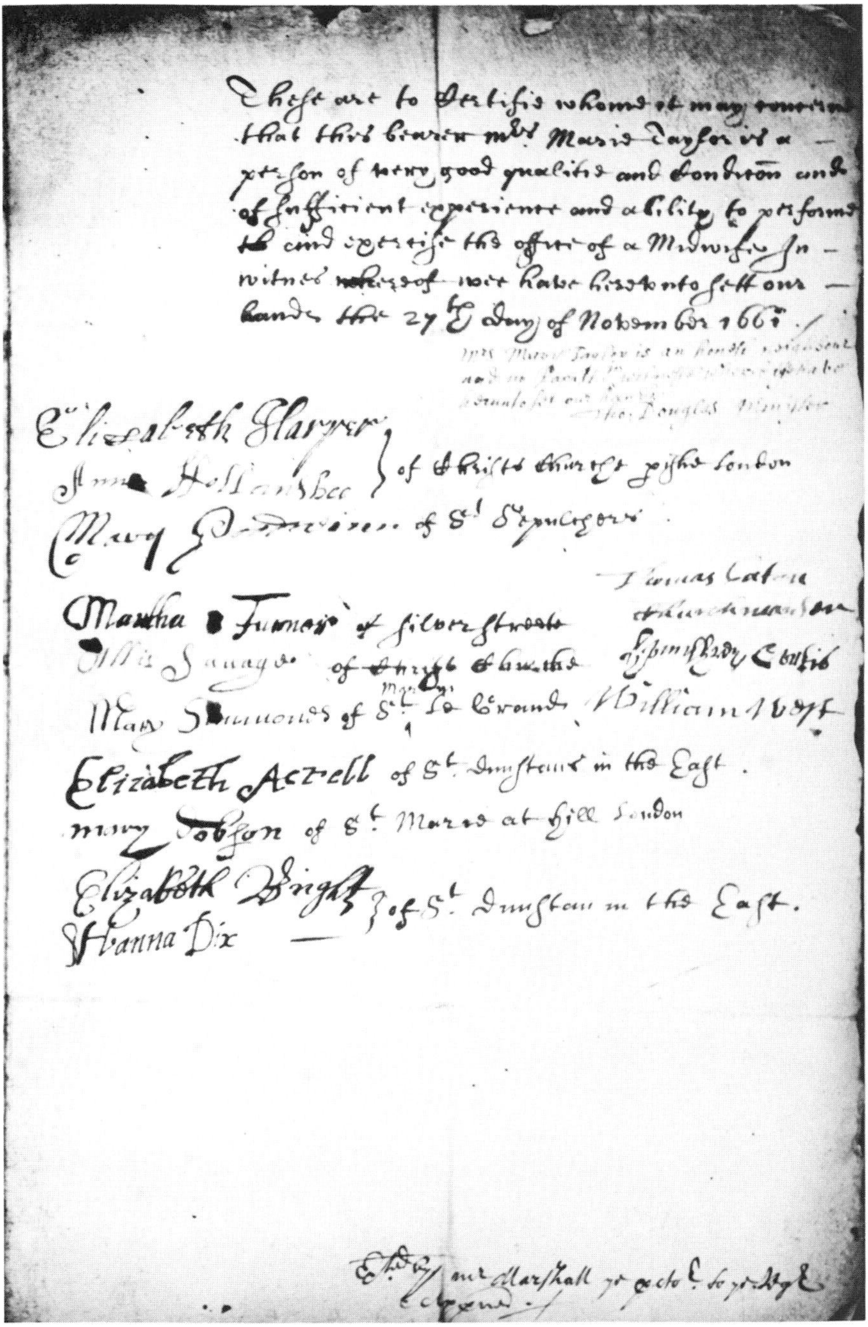

These are to certifie whome it may concerne that this bearer Mrs Marie Tayler is a person of very good qualitie and condition and of sufficient experience and ability to performe and exercise the office of a Midwife In witnes whereof wee have hereunto sett our hands this 27th day of November 1661.

Mrs Marie Tayler is an honest [illegible] [illegible] hereunto set our hands Tho: Douglas Minister

Elizabeth Harper, Anne Hollandbee } of Christs church parishe London

Mary [illegible] of St Sepulchers

Thomas Caton churchwarden

Martha Turner of Silver Streete

Alice Savage of [illegible]

Mary Simmonds of St Martins le Grand William [illegible]

Elizabeth Acrell of St Dunstans in the East.

Mary Dobson of St Maries at hill London

Elizabeth Wright, Hanna Dix } of St Dunstan in the East.

[illegible] Mr Marshall [illegible]

Plate 3. Midwife's license. In this case the witnesses are from several different parishes.

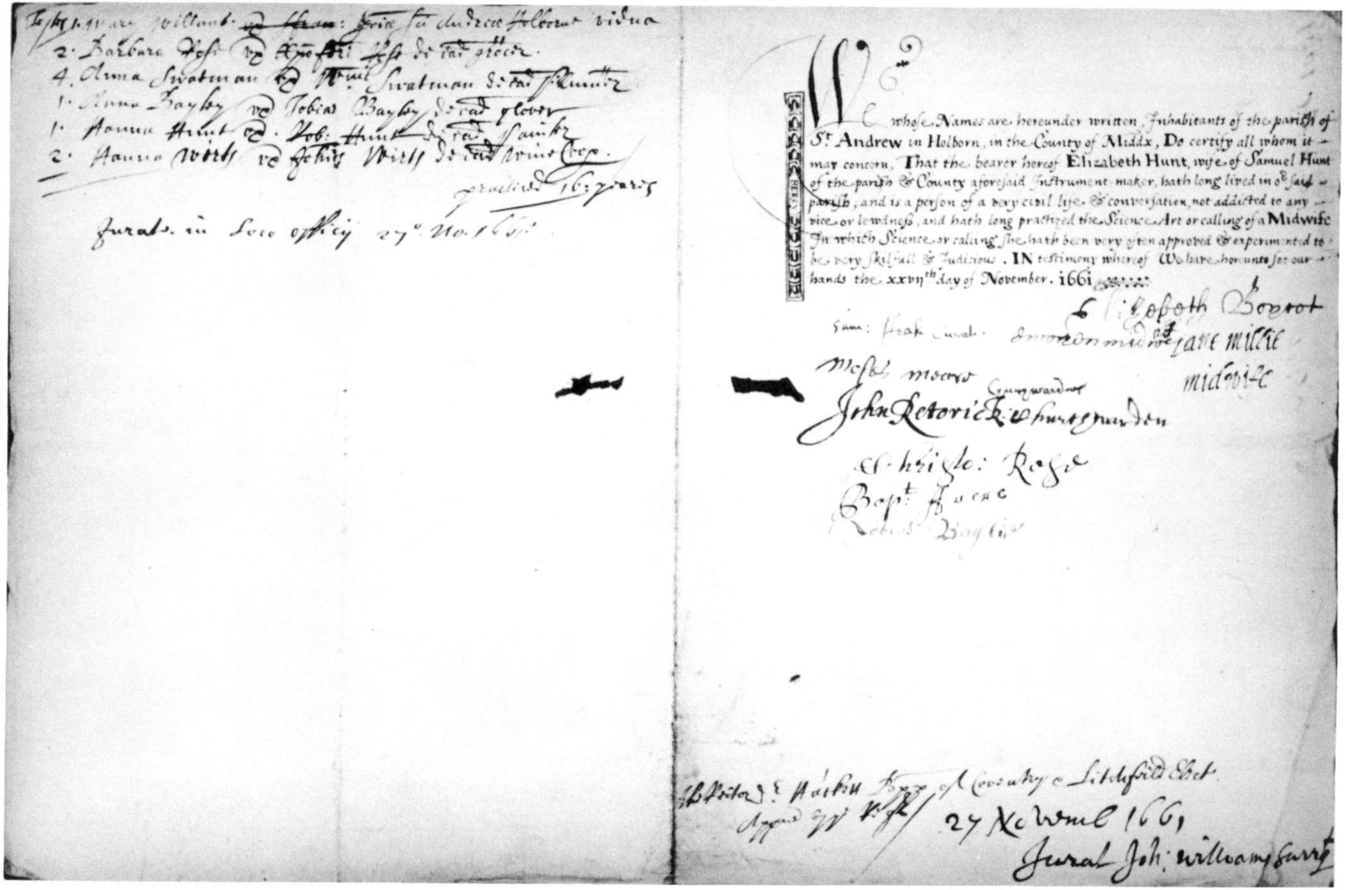

We whose Names are hereunder written, Inhabitants of the parish of St Andrew in Holborn, in the County of Middx, Do certify all whom it may concern, That the bearer hereof Elizabeth Hunt, wife of Samuel Hunt of the parish & County aforesaid Instrument maker, hath long lived in o^r said parish; and is a person of a very civil life & conversation, not addicted to any vice or lewdness, and hath long practized the Science Art or calling of a Midwife In which Science or calling she hath been very often approved & experimented to be very skilfull & Judicious. IN testimony whereof We have hereunto set our hands the xxvii^th day of November. 1661

Jane Millie midwife

John Retorick Churchwarden

Plate 4. Midwife's license. Such careful engrossing was unusual. Note that midwifery is referred to as a "Science Art or calling."

Wee whose names are hereunder written doe briefly certify unto all whom it may concern, That Mrs Debora Bromfield is a person who has long practized ye skill of Midwivery, with good success: And being one of an orderly & sober conversacion, & well affected to ye Doctrine & Discipline of the Church of England, & being singularly well qualified for ye imploymt of a midwife, wee humbly recomend her to be continued therein. Given under or hands ye 22th. day of May. 1662.

Tho: Exton

Being credibly informed of what is here affected, I doe verily beleive the truth thereof, and therefore iudge her fitt (with submission to Authorytie) to be continued in the imployment of a Midwife.

James Lambe Rector of St Andrewes Holb. Lond.

Sam: ffirth Cur. St Andw.

John Petowck;
Churchwarden.

1o Augt 1662.
Conceedatur Licentia
Rich: Chaworth.

Debora Bromfield

---

§ Plate 5. Midwife's license. Thomas Exton's florid signature appears on a number of licenses; he either signed the character statement, as here, or granted the license. The name of Richard Chaworth, who approved this license, is also familiar.

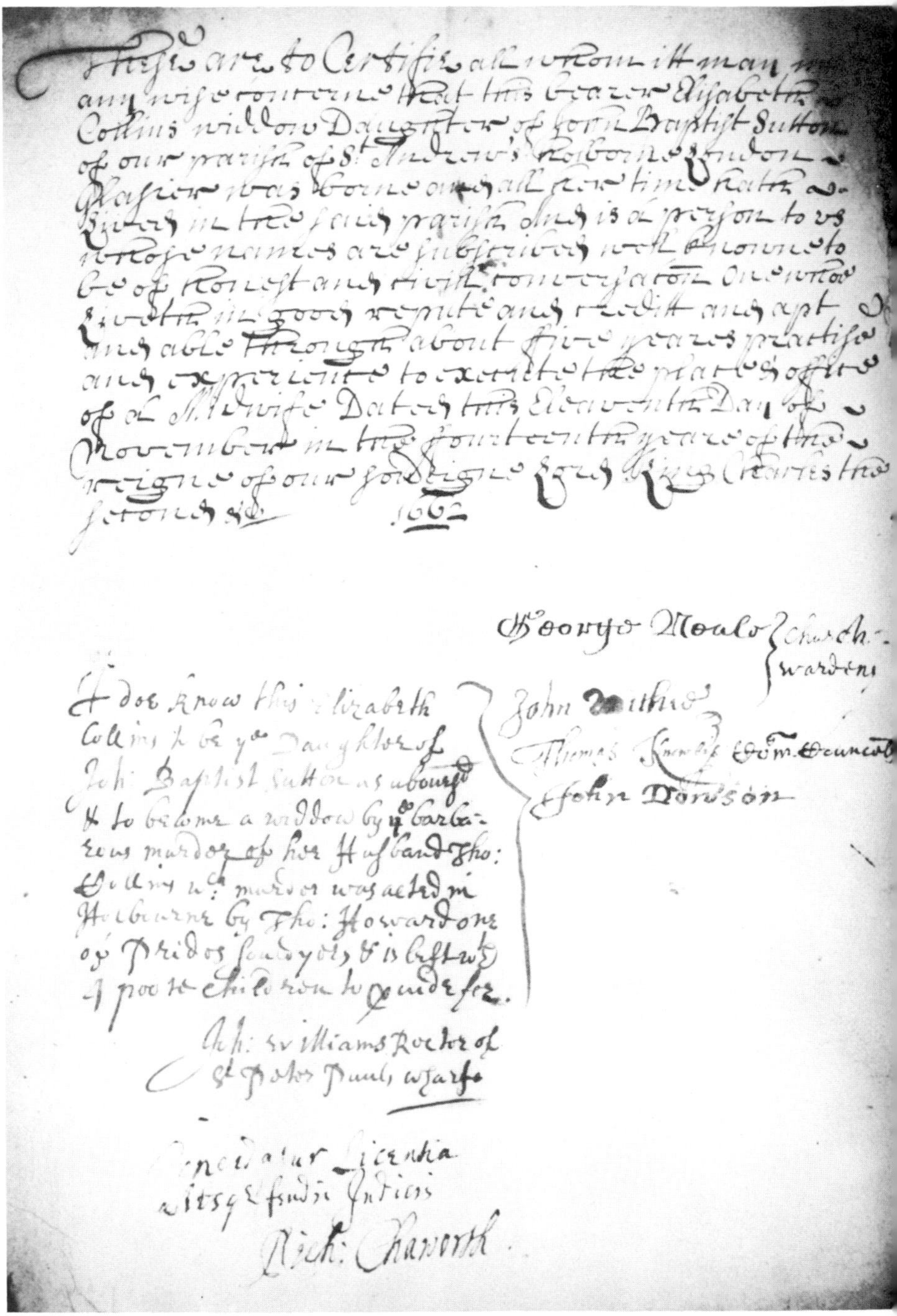
These are to Certifie all whom itt may any wise concerne that this bearer Elizabeth Collins widdow Daughter of John Baptist Sutton of our parish of St. Andrew's Holborne London Glasier was borne and all her time hath lived in the said parish And is a person to us whose names are subscribed well knowne to be of honest and civill conversation One who liveth in good repute and credit and apt and able through about five yeares practise and experience to execute the place & office of a Midwife Dated this Eleaventh Day of November in the fourteenth yeare of the reigne of our soveraigne Lord King Charles the second &c 1662

George Moule } Churchwardens

John Dowson

I doe know this Elizabeth Collins to be ye Daughter of Joh: Baptist Sutton as above sd & to become a widdow by ye barbarous murder of her Husband Tho: Collins wch murder was acted in Holbourne by Tho: Howard one of Pride's souldyers & is left wth 4 poore children to pvide for.

Joh: Williams Rector of St Peter Paul's wharfe

Concedatur Licentia

Rich: Chaworth

Plate 6. Midwife's license. Rector John Williams says of the applicant: "I doe know th Elizabeth Collins to be ye Daughter of Joh: Baptist Sutton as above sd [said] & to become widdow by ye barbarous murder of her Husband Tho: Collins wch murder was acted i Holbourne by Tho: Howard one of Pride's souldyers & is left wth 4 poore children to pvic for." Col. Thomas Pride, of Pride's Purge, was a regicide.

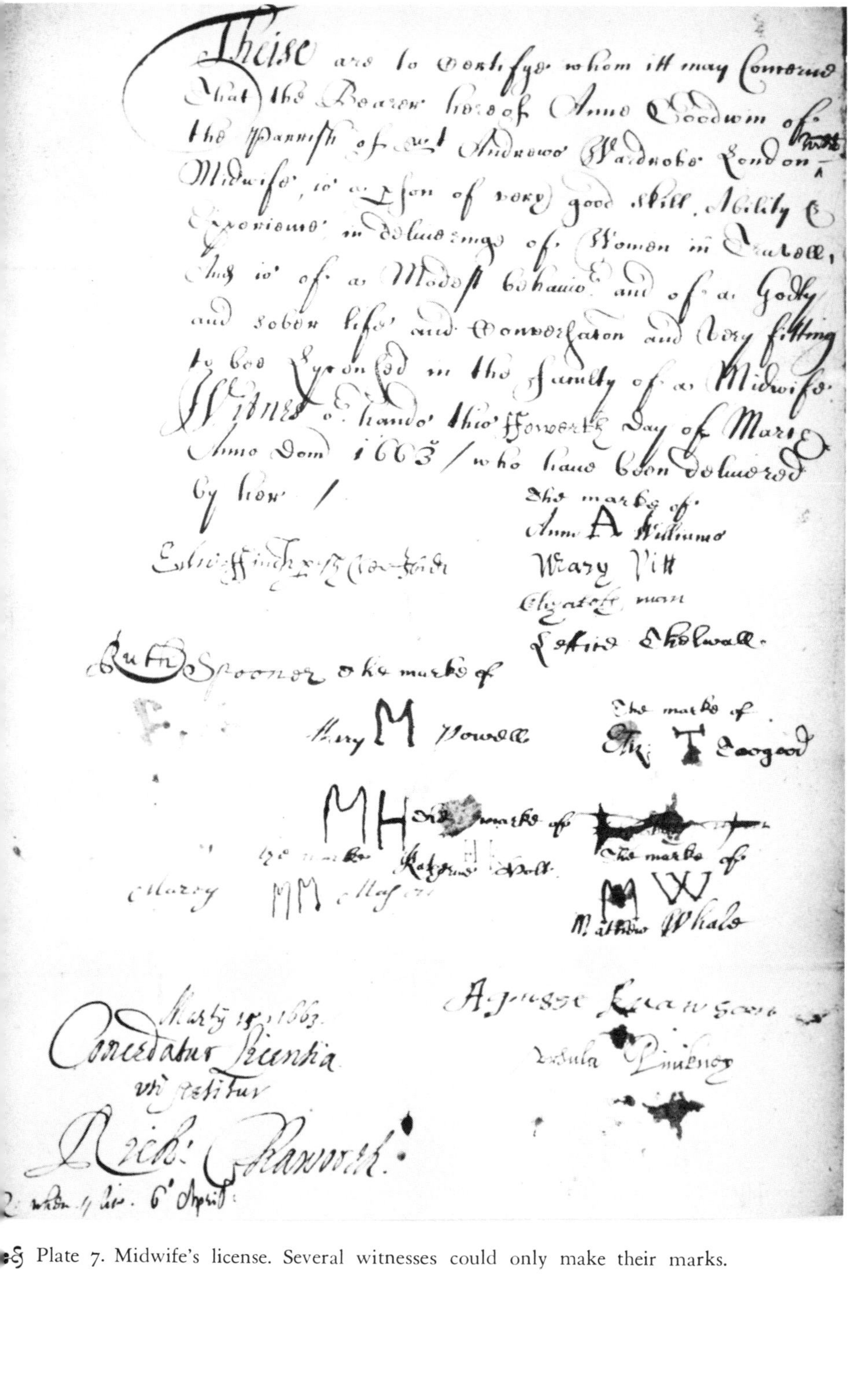

Plate 7. Midwife's license. Several witnesses could only make their marks.

≈§ Plate 8. Midwife's license. "These are to certifye that Anne Gill is a person able t undertake the office of Midwife. And allsoe y^t [that] shee is Loyall to ye Kinge & conform able to the Doctrine & Discipline of the church of England. In witness whereof six wome whome she hath safe delivered of children have subscribed theyr names & the parson an churchwardens of Barnet." Barnet, East Barnet, and High Barnet are near London.

wifery. She was also separately examined in this subject by eight women, presumably experienced midwives.[4]

The midwife was also required to take an oath of office before she could be licensed. The oath administered at Canterbury to Eleonor Pead speaks for itself.

> I, Eleonor Pead, admitted to the office and occupation of a midwife, will faithfully and diligently exercise the said office according to such cunning and knowledge as God hath given me: and that I will be ready to help and aid as well poor as rich women being in labor and travail of child, and will always be ready both to poor and rich, in exercising and executing of my said office. Also, I will not permit or suffer that woman being in labour or travail shall name any other to be the father of her child, than only he who is the right and true father thereof; and that I will not suffer any other body's child to be set, brought, or laid before any woman delivered of child in the place of her natural child, so far forth as I can know and understand. Also, I will not use any kind of sorcery or incantation in the time of the travail of any woman; and that I will not destroy the child born of any woman, nor cut, nor pull off the head thereof, or otherwise dismember or hurt the same, or suffer it to be so hurt or dismembered, by any manner of ways or means. Also, that in the ministration of the sacrament of baptism in the time of necessity I will use apt and the accustomed words of the same sacrament, that is to say, these words following, or the like in effect; *I christen thee in the name of the Father, the Son, and the Holy Ghost,* and none other profane words. And that in such time of necessity, in baptizing any infant born, and pouring water upon the head of the same infant, I will use pure and clean water, and not any rose or damask water, or water made of any confection or mixture: and that I will certify the curate of the parish church of every such baptizing. [Strype, 1824]

An oath taken by midwives in 1584 at the direction of the Bishop of Chester specified that they not use "any witchcraft, charms, relics or invocation to any Saint in the time of travail" (Raines, 1853).

A *Book of Oaths* of office for many kinds of officials, high and low, which was issued in 1649 (Anon.) includes an "Oath that is to be ministered to a Mid-wife by the Bishop or his Chancellor of the

---

4. Anon. (1895), Blencowe (1851), Burn (1797), Thompson and Frere (1928).

Diocese, when she is licensed to exercise that Office of a Midwife." The restrictions of the oath in effect are a catalogue of the abuses of midwifery at that period.

You shall sweare, First, that you shall be diligent and faithfull, and readie to helpe every Woman labouring of Childe, as well the poore as the riche; and that in time of nessitie [sic], you shall not forsake or leave the poore woman, to go to the Rich.

2. Item, Yee shall neither cause nor suffer any, woman to name, or put any other Father to the Childe, but onely him which is the very true Father thereof indeed.

3. Item, you shall not suffer any woman to pretend, faine, or surmize herselfe to be delivered of a Childe, who is not indeed; neither to claime any other womans Childe for her owne.

4. Item, you shall not suffer any Womans Childe to be murthered, maymed, or otherwise hurt, as much as you may; and so often as you shall perceive any perill or jeopardie, either in the Woman, or in the Childe, in any such wise, as you shall bee in doubt what shall chance thereof, you shal thenceforth in due time send for other Midwifes and expert women in that facultie, and use their advice and counsell in that behalfe.

5. Item, that you shall not in any wise use or exercise any manner of Witchcraft, Charme; or Sorcery, Invocation, or other Prayers than may stand with Gods Laws and the Kings.

6. Item, you shall not give any counsell, or minister any Herbe, Medicine, or Potion, or any other thing, to any Woman being with Childe whereby she should destroy or cast out that she goeth withal before her time.

7. Item, You shall not enforce any Woman being with childe by any paine, or by any ungodly wayes or meanes, to give you any more for your paines or labour in bringing her a [i.e. to] bed, then they would otherwise do.

8. Item, you shall not consent, agree, give, or keepe counsell, that any woman be delivered secretly of that which she goeth with, but in the presence of two or three lights readie.

9. Item, you shall be secret, and not open any matter appertaining to your Office in the presence of any man, unlesse necessity or great urgent cause do constraine you so to do.

10. Item, if any childe bee dead borne, you your selfe shall see it

buried in such secret place as neither Hogg nor Dogg, nor any other Beast may come unto it, and in such sort done, as it may not be found or perceived, as much as you may; And that you shall not suffer any such childe to be cast into the Jaques or any other inconvenient place.

11. Item, If you shall know any Midwife using or doing any thing contrary to any of the premisses, or in any other wise than shall be seemely or convenient, you shall forthwith detect open to shew the same to me,[5] or my Chancellor for the time being.

12. Item, you shall use your selfe in honest behaviour unto the woman being lawfully admitted to the roome [station, rank] and Office of a Midwife in all things accordingly.

13. Item, That you shall truly present to my selfe, or my Chancellor, all such women as you shall know from time to time to occupie and exercise the roome of a Midwife within my foresaid Diocesse and jurisdiction of *A*.[6] without my License and admission.

14. Item, you shall not make or assigne any Deputie or Deputies to exercise or occupie under you in your absence the Office or roome of a Midwife, but such as you shall perfectly know to be of right honest and discreet behaviour, as also apt, able, & having sufficient knowledge and experience to exercise the said roome and Office.

15. Item, you shall not bee Privie, or consent, that any Priest, or other partie, shall in your absence, or in your companie, or of your knowledge or sufferance, Baptise any child, by any Masse, Latine Service, or Prayers, then such as are appointed by the Lawes of the Church of *Englande;* neither shall you consent, that any child, born by any woman, who shall be delivered by you, shall be carried away without being Baptised in the Parish by the Ordinarie Minister, where the said child is borne, unless it be in the case of necessitie, Baptised privately, according to the Booke of Common Prayer: but you shall forthwith upon understanding thereof, either give knowledge to me the said Bishop, or my Chancellour for the time being. All of which Articles and Charge you shall faithfully observe and keepe, so help you God and by the contents of this Booke.[7]

It was the custom for a bishop to make periodic visits for inspection

5. The bishop.
6. This probably means that the name of the appropriate diocese should be inserted here.
7. Presumably this was the Bible upon which the oath was taken.

of the churches in his diocese. During such visitations he inquired not only into the spiritual well-being of his flock and the physical condition of the church building but granted an occasional license, collected fees for licenses [8] already in force, and issued numerous instructions to the clergy and churchwardens. These instructions, or "injunctions," have been preserved from as early as 1537. Typically it was specified that "all curates must openly in the church, teach and instruct the midwives of the very words and form of baptism" (Frere and Kennedy, 1910). The "Articles of Visitation," that is, the questions to be asked on the occasion of an episcopal visit of inspection, which were drawn up in 1554 by Edmund Bonner, Bishop of London, are quite detailed (Cardwell, 1844). Article I asks whether, other than in an emergency, any woman is acting as a midwife who has not been examined and admitted to office by the bishop or his representative. Article II inquires whether authorized midwives are "catholic [9] and faithful, discreet and sober, diligent and ready to help" all who seek them. Article III asks if midwives use "any witchcraft, charms, sorcery, invocations," etc. Article IV pertains to baptism. Article VI inquires if "there be any other disorder or evil behaviour" among the midwives, their assistants, or their patients. The "Interrogatories and Demands" of John Hooper, Bishop of Worchester, in 1552 were equally concerned with the correct form of baptism, but according to the dictates of the Reformation [10] (Nevinson, 1852).

At another visitation in 1559, made in this case by representatives of Queen Elizabeth I, it was asked, "Whether you knowe anye that doe use charmes, sorcerye, enchauntments, inuocations, circles, witchcrafts, soothsayinge, or any lyke craftes or ymaginations inuented by the Devyll and specyallye in the tyme of women's travayle" (Pettigrew, 1844). A similar question was asked among the "Articles to be enquired of, within the Province of Canterburie, in the Metropoliticall visitation of the most reuerende father in God, Edmonde Archbishop of

8. Information is scanty regarding the amount of the fee for the license. It is recorded that the wife of William Silke, surgeon, paid 18s.6d. in 1662 for her license as midwife; her husband's license cost 13s. 6d. (Hurd-Mead, 1938). Fees, not necessarily typical, for midwives' licenses were 1s or 2s. in 1706 (Barnes, 1903; Williams, 1901), 17s.6d. between 1709 and 1719 (Kerslake, 1850), 8 guineas in 1714, 3s.4d. in 1719, and £10 in 1738 (Hurd-Mead, 1938).

9. Bishop Bonner's diocese was in the Roman Catholic province of Thomas Cranmer, Archbishop of Canterbury.

10. Bishop Hooper had left the Catholic Church to join the Protestants.

Canterburie, Primate of all Englande, and Metropolitane" in 1576 (Nicholson, 1843). Richard Barnes, Bishop of Durham, left the record of "Certeyne Monicions and Iniunctions given . . . on Tewesdaie the first daie of October 1577." Item 8 read, in part,

> And we charge and commaunde yow duly, from tyme to tyme, to present the names and surnames of all suche women as shall taike in hande, or enterprice, to babtize, or at the childes birthe use supersticious ceremonyes, orizons, charmes, or develishe rytes or sorceries.[11]

Many other visitation articles asked similar questions.[12]

Midwives practicing without a license or otherwise violating professional rules could be "presented," that is, charged before an ecclesiastical court, brought to trial, and fined or otherwise punished.[13] Two presentments on the fabric rolls of York Minster for the period between 1362 and 1550 (Raine, 1859) read in translation:

> Driffield parva. . . . Agnes Marshall, alias Saunder of Emeswell, exercises the office of midwife without having either experience or knowledge of midwifery; moreover, she uses incantations.

> Alne. . . . Item, Agnes Hobson of Alne administers love potions or apothecaries' potions of her own preparation, wherewith she destroys the foetus in the womb and even the mother, and she has given the said potions to very many women. She has made expiation 2 July.[14]

11. Another part of the same injunction from Bishop Barnes, a Protestant, reveals doctrine regarding the fate of the souls of infants dying unbaptized: "And that yowe hereof admonishe your parishioners, and therewithall also teache them, that, if any infant dye without publique babtisme first to it ministred, that the same is not to be condemned or adiuged as a damned sowle, but to be well hoped of, and the body to be interred in the churche yearde, yet without ringinge or any divine service or solemnity, bycause the same was not solemnly professed and receyved into the church and congregacion."

12. Anon. (1864), Aveling (1872), Brinkworth (1947), Cardwell (1844), Frere (1910), Frere and Kennedy (1910), Kinloch (1848), Owen and Blakeway (1825), Raine (1850).

13. Atkinson (1907), Burn (1797), Kittredge (1929), Williams (1901). The jurisdiction of a spiritual court over such an offense was successfully challenged on at least one occasion: "If there be a suit in the spiritual court, against a woman for exercising the trade of a midwife without license of the ordinary [an archbishop, a bishop, or his deputy], against the canons: a prohibition lieth [is sustainable]: for this is not any spiritual function, of which they have cognisance. 2 *Roll's Abr. 286*" (Burn, 1797; Godolphin, 1687).

14. This charge does not state that the woman was a midwife, but the context suggests this was her profession.

From the Bampton churchwardens' presentments for 1691: "We do present Elizabeth Harrison for acting as a midwife without a licence, to the prejudice of several persons" (M.N., 1900).

For the archdeaconry of Buckingham a whole series of presentments in 1662 has been set down. Brinkworth, the editor of these important transcripts, gives the clues for interpretation of the Latin abbreviations:

> (Deanery of Burnham) p. the wife of John Church, midwife without supra ["approbacion or license," previously mentioned] 17 Oct. 62: comp. et iurata ad exequendum officium obstetricis etc. [Presentment: the wife of John Church, midwife without sanction or license. She appeared and took the oath to practice as a midwife, etc.] Chesham. . . . One goodwife Warde, a midwife. 17 Oct. 62: qu. etc. pco. comp. et iurata ad exequendum officium obstetricis. [Added in margin of original] dimittitur. [17 Oct. 1662 was sought, etc. Public proclamation having been made, she appeared and was sworn for exercise of the office of midwife. Case dismissed.]

In Turfield Joane Munday was presented on 4 December 1662 for practicing midwifery "(for ought wee knowe) without a licence." Jane, wife of John Drewce of Aylesbury, was presented for the same offense on 24 September 1662, was cited on 10 October, failed to appear, and was excommunicated. This appears to have been a not unusual penalty. The names of a good many midwives are followed by a date and the terse notation "c., pco., non comp., ex."—*citata, praeconizatio facta, non comparuit, excommunicatur* (having been cited and public proclamation having been made, she did not appear, and is excommunicated) (Brinkworth, 1947).

In the London County Record Office are lists of schoolteachers, surgeons, and midwives who were presented at the Consistory Court of London for violations. A great many of the errant midwives were either excommunicated or fined.

An amusing letter was written on 2 October 1675 by a clergyman, Benjamin Younge, to Dr. Thomas Exton, Vicar General to Humphrey, Bishop of London. The letter, addressed to Exton at his lodgings in Doctors' Commons and now in the license collection at the Guildhall Library, intercedes for one Dennys Younge. Dennys, perhaps a relative of the Reverend Mr. Younge, was supposed to be excommunicated for practicing midwifery without a license. It was her second offense. Mr. Younge intercedes tactfully in this matter:

> An Excomunication from yor Officer against two Midwifes practicing in my Parish without Licēncēs. I presumed to forber denouncing of it till I had dealt with them to submit to ye authority of ye Court and to take out Licēnēs of practice. Accordingly the barer hereof Dennys Younge . . . hath so far been ruled by me, as to come to yo^u to crave license of practice. Shee is a woman skillful in that way as hath been often approved, & ye very citation grants: but her skill hath been most comonly made use of by ye poorer people from whom she received very little or no advantage, which made me bold the last year to sollicit your favor to her, when the like excomunication came to me against her, which yō were pleased to grant me. . . . I humbly beg ye favor of you, yf shee may be dispatcht with speed, & at as cheap a rate as may be, because her circumstances are but ordinary, & her practice inconsiderable. . . . I am willing to think that this is ye most acceptable way of executing your orders, which may be done upon most people but ye Quakers who are stubborn and refractory. Other persons will be likely to submit more easily when they shall hear yt [that] they may be used mildly and gently. This Sir with my most humble Duty to my Reverend Diocesan, my faithfull respects and obedience to your selfe, is all from
>
> S^r Yo^r most humble Servt
Ben: Younge

I am glad to report that Dr. Exton granted the license on 4 October.

In 1616, or perhaps a little earlier, the Chamberlen family became involved with the midwives. The story has been told in detail by Aveling and others, and will only be summarized here. William Chamberlen the obstetrician had two sons, *both* named Peter, who took up their father's profession. In 1616 the midwives of the City of London petitioned the King for permission to incorporate into a society. The petition, which had the support of both Peter Chamberlens, pointed out the urgent need for better training of midwives through "lectures upon Anatomies and other Aucthorety for orders and helpes for instruccon and increase of skill amongst them." The College of Physicians, to which the petition was referred, agreed that reforms were greatly to be desired but opposed the formation of a corporation. The College suggested that before the midwives were licensed

> by the Bisshopp or his Chauncellour they be first examined and approved by the President of the College of the Phisitions and two or iij of the gravest of that Society such as the President shall nominate. And likewise for abuses and disorders by any of them comytted thay may be censured of the Colledge accordinge as ys used in all other evell practizers in Phissick. And for the bettringe of their skill and knowledge the College maketh offer to dispute such grave and learned men as shall allwaies be ready to resolve all their doubts and instruct them in what they desire concerninge Midwiferye and once or twice in the yeare to make privat dissections and Annattomyes to the use of their whole Company.

Peter Chamberlen III, son of Peter Chamberlen the Younger, was a Fellow of the College of Physicians and a successful obstetrician. In 1633 he attempted himself to organize the midwives and, according to an angry contemporary account, to secure sole authority to instruct, approve, and license them. His proposal so disturbed the midwives that they petitioned the King and the College of Physicians to prevent Chamberlen from being allowed to gain control over the profession. The College took the side of the midwives, and Chamberlen's project failed. In 1634 the midwives again petitioned, this time for permission to incorporate. The Chamberlen family had continued its support, but effective opposition came from the organized medical profession, and the petition was denied.[15]

The original recommendation of the College of Physicians, however, was implemented in 1642 when authority to license midwives was transferred from the bishops to the physicians and surgeons at Surgeons' Hall. This was an important advance. A good many years later, Elizabeth Cellier set down her version of the ensuing period:

> The Physicians and Chirurgions contending about it [the role of the midwife at a delivery], it was adjudged a Chyrurgical Operation, and the Midwives were Licensed at *Chirurgion's Hall, but not till they had passed three Examinations, before six skilful Midwives, and as many Chirurgions expert in the Art of Midwifery*. Thus it continued until the Act of Uniformity passed, which sent the Mid-

15. Anon. (1895), Aveling (1872, 1882), Goodall (1684), Spencer (1927).

wives back to *Doctors Commons,* where they pay their money (*take an Oath which is impossible for them to keep*) and return home as skilful as they went thither.

I make no reflections on those learned Gentlemen the Licensers, but refer the curious for their further satisfaction, to the Yearly Bills of Mortality, from [16]42 to [16]62: Collections of which they may find at *Clerks-Hall:* Which if they please to compare with these of late Years, they will find there did not then happen the eight [sic] part of the Casualties, either to Women or Children, as do now. [Celleor, 1687]

In June, 1687, Mrs. Cellier submitted a petition to James II (Oldys, 1809). In this remarkable document she proposed the founding of a royal hospital, to be maintained by a corporation of a thousand skilled, dues-paying midwives. Unfortunately, as Aveling (1872) points out, it appears that the scheme was far from practical and that it would have been operated in large measure for the financial benefit of Mrs. Cellier. It is regrettable, however, that the plan for professional instruction of midwives was not implemented. As it was, licensing, which had gone "back to Doctors Commons," that is, to routine ecclesiastical regulation, was to remain there for many years. Even the oath of office, if one is to believe the vehement Mrs. Cellier, could not be kept.

The Norwich Diocese Book and records at Somerset House note the issuing of numerous licenses. Examples read, in translation: "Wells, Mary, 26 September [1662]. License to Mary Wells, midwife, wife of Thomas Wells of the Parish of Bletchingly." "Taylor, Jane. 9 April 1663. A license was granted to her as, midwife in the parish of St. Olaf, Southwark." There are records of midwives being licensed by the Kirk Session of Perth in 1611, by the Register of St. Finn Barrs Cathedral, Cork, in 1685 and 1686, and by the King and Queen's College of Physicians in Ireland in 1696.[16]

Although ecclesiastical licensing of qualified midwives probably began soon after 1512, I have not come across the text of a license issued in the sixteenth or first half of the seventeenth century. The Guildhall Library has a fine collection of original licenses granted to residents of various London parishes (see Plates 1–8) and there are others in Lambeth Palace. Mrs. Cellier was in error when she said that licensing by the Church was resumed in 1662; perhaps she had forgotten the

16. Barnes (1903), Bax (1893), R.C. (1861), Ringland (1870), Wallace-James (1900), Williams (1901).

correct date by the time she wrote her account in 1687. Episcopal licenses in the Guildhall collection date from January 1660. An unusually detailed example, issued 16 November 1661, reads in part:

> These are to certifie the hono^ble the Consistory court of the Lord Bishop of London held by the right worp^ll Doctor Richard Chaworth his Chancellor in the Hall of Doctors Commons that Judith Newman wife of William Newman of the parish of Allhallows the less hath lived in the said parish thirty yeares and upwards during which tyme shee hath demeaned herself honestly and in love and charity with her neighbours, And that shee is in our judgments able and sufficient for the Office and ffunction of a Midwife which shee hath many yeares past been exercised in, And therefore we Recomend her unto yr honor for the exercise of such an office and ffunction.

Appended are the signatures of the curate, two churchwardens, two "common counsellmen," and one midwife and the mark of another. There is also a list of six women, presumably delivered by Judith Newman. Under the list is the statement *approbat et Jurat testes et obstetrix* [sic] *pro Mr. Joh: Williams Surrogat in Loco Registri 16 Novemb. 1661* and, in another hand, "practised 15 or 16 yeares." [17]

The Guildhall licenses vary somewhat in form. In general, there is a statement, usually in a clear hand, that the bearer, a resident of a specified parish of London, is a woman of honest life and "conversation" (demeanor). Frequently it is added that she is a member of, or conformable to, the Church of England. There may also be an assertion that she is an experienced or competent midwife. The testimonial certificate is signed by the minister, rector, or curate of the parish and often by two churchwardens. Usually the names of three to six or eight other men and women also are listed as witnesses. The names of the parishes of residence and the occupations of the witnesses or their husbands (instrument maker, cordwainer, tailor, upholsterer, etc.) may be given. Occasionally a witness is identified as a midwife. Since the names of the witnesses are all appended in the same handwriting rather than as actual signatures, it seems likely that illiteracy was not unusual. Often included is a separate list of the names of six women, their husbands' names, and their parishes. Before the name of each

17. The surrogate in the Church of England was the deputy of the bishop or of his chancellor.

woman appears the numeral 1, 2, 3, or 4. Presumably this is a list of women delivered by the applicant and the number of confinements involved.

At the bottom of the parchment is the license proper, a statement in Latin to the effect that on a specified date the applicant appeared before, and was approved and sworn by, a person who signs the statement as a surrogate. Often the witnesses also were sworn. The legal formula varies, even as written by the same surrogate. It might read *Margarita Corney jurat 12 Nov. 1661 coram M*ro [*Magistro*] *Jo: Wms Sur.*to [*Williams Surrogato*] [18] or *22 Martii 1675 Anna Dobson et mulieres pecia* [*paroecia,* parish] *jurat*[*a*] *cor*[*am*] *me Tho: Exton.*[19] Sometimes *ffiat Licentia* or *Concedatur Licentia* [20] is added.

To modern eyes the striking feature of these documents is that the principal, and sometimes the only, mentioned qualification of the midwife was that she was a person of good character. If there was any reference to her professional competence, it was usually to the number of years that she had functioned as a midwife, although laymen sometimes testified to her skill. Thus, like her training, the licensing of the midwife was seriously inadequate by modern standards. Nevertheless, there did develop during the sixteenth and seventeenth centuries a procedure for admitting to the licensed practice of midwifery only those women who were respected in their parishes for their morality, discretion, and sobriety and for their experience in their craft. On the long path to effective regulation, it was not a bad beginning.

18. Margaret Corney took the oath 12 November 1661 in the presence of Master John Williams, Surrogate.
19. (22 March 1675 Anna Dobson and women of the parish took the oath in my presence. Thomas Exton.)
20. (Let the license be granted.)

Bibliography

Abbott, G. F. 1903. *Macedonian Folklore.* Cambridge, University Press, pp. 106, 139.

Ackermann, A. S. E. 1923. *Popular Fallacies Explained and Corrected.* . . . London, Old Westminster Press, pp. 71, 72.

Adams, F. D. 1938. *The Birth and Development of the Geological Sciences.* London, Baillière, Tindall and Cox, pp. 98–102.

Adams, Francis. 1849. *The Genuine Works of Hippocrates.* . . . London, The Sydenham Society, *2,* 745.

Addy, S. A. 1888. *A Glossary of Words Used in the Neighbourhood of Sheffield.* London, Trübner, pp. 302, 328.

Adelmann, H. B. 1942. *The Embryological Treatises of Hieronymus Fabricius ab Aquapendente.* Ithaca, N.Y., Cornell University Press, pp. 152, 248, 270, 366, 747, 765.

Aelianus, Claudius. 1744. *De natura animalium.* . . . London, Gulielmus Bowyer, Lib. III, cap. XVII; Lib. XIV, cap. XVIII.

Aetius. 1543. *Contractae ex ueteribus medicinae sermones XVI.* Venetiis, Farrea, pp. 74–75.

Agricola, Georgius. 1657. *De natura fossilium.* Basileae, Emanuelis König, pp. 603, 612, 615.

Agrippa, H. C. 1651. *Three Books of Occult Philosophy.* . . . London, R. W. for Gregory Moule, pp. 82–83.

A. H. 1881. Medical folk-lore: an 'eagle stone.' *Notes and Queries,* 6th ser., *3,* 327.

Albarel, P. 1924. L'Oraison de sainte Marguerite, pour les femmes en couche. *Chron. méd., 31,* 231–33.

Albertus Magnus. 1542. *Libellus de formatione hominis.* Antverpiae [cited by Iversen, 1939].

——— 1569. *De mineralibus et rebus metallicis.* . . . Coloniae, apud Ioannem Birckmannum & Theodorum Baumium, Lib. II, cap. V.

——— 1580. *De secretis mulierum libellus.* . . . [no place, no pub.], cap. VII, VIII.

——— 1581. *Daraus man alle Heimligkeit.* . . . Franckfurt am Mayn, Johann Schmidt, p. 3.

——— 1637. *The Secrets of Albertus Magnus. Of the Vertues of Herbes, Stones, and Certaine Beasts.* London, T. Cotes [no pagination].

Aldrovandus, Vlyssis. 1648. *Mvsaeum metallicvm.* . . . Bononiae [no pub.], pp. 580–90.

Amabille, G. 1937. La valore delle reazione de Davis con estratto testiculare per la diagnosi prenatale di sesso. *Clin. ostet. ginec., 39,* 204–09.

Ammannus, Paulus. 1675. *Brevis ad materiam medicam in usum philiatrorum manuductio.* Lipsiae, Christianus Michaelis, *3,* 17–18.

Amoureux. 1771. Lettre. Réponse par de la Brousse. *J. méd. chir. pharm. (Paris), 36,* 217–27, 227–33.

——— 1772. Seconde lettre. . . . *J. méd. chir. pharm. (Paris), 38,* 62–76.

Andrews, E. A., ed. 1907. *A New Latin Dictionary. Harper's Latin Dictionary,* New York, American Book Co.

Andrews, Edmund. 1947. A History of Scientific English. New York, R. R. Smith, p. 39.

[Anon.] [1530?] *Eyn unterricht für die hebammen / wie sie in der not Tauffen sollen* [no place, no pub.].

[Anon.] 1649. *The Book of Oaths, and the Severall Forms Thereof, Both Antient and Modern.* . . . London, W. Lee, M. Walbancke, D. Pakeman, and G. Bedle, pp. 284–90.

[Anon.] 1684. *A Collection of Articles, Injunctions, Canons, Orders, Ordinances, and Constitutions Ecclesiastical, with Other Publick Records of the Church of England.* . . . London, Blanch Pawlet, pp. 175–82.

[Anon.] 1739. *Hochfürstliche Wirzburgische Hebammen-Ordnung.* Wirzburg, M. A. Engmann.

[Anon.] 1773. *Dictionnaire raisonné-universel de matière médicale.* . . . Paris, P. F. Didot, *6,* 80.

[Anon.] 1811. Interesting Horse Cause. Tried at the Oakham Assizes, Friday, July 26, before Mr. Baron Thompson. Franey v. Fancourt. *Sporting Mag., 38,* 209–14.

[Anon.] 1817. *The Statutes of the Realm. Printed by Command of His Majesty King George the Third.* . . . [no place, no pub.].

[Anon.] 1840. *Ancient Laws and Institutes of England.* . . . *Also, Monumenta ecclesiastica.* . . . [no place, no pub.].

[Anon.] 1887. The free martin. *Brit. med. J., 1,* 43, 93, 141, 187.

[Anon.] 1895. Celebrated midwives of the 17th and beginning of the 18th centuries: With a short account of the present position of midwives. *St Thom. Hosp. Gaz. (London), 5,* 33–36.

[Anon.] 1899. An obstetrical charm. *Medical Age (Detroit), 17,* 61.

[Anon.] 1899. Cauls. *Lancet, 1,* 137.

[Anon.] 1956. Antenatal sexing. *Lancet, 270,* 195–96.

Aristotle. 1910. *Historia animalium.* Oxford, Clarendon Press, Book VI, 18, 572^a; Book VI, 22, 577^a; Book VIII, 24, 605^a.

Aristotle [pseud.] 1782. *Complete and Experienced Midwife.* . . . London [no pub.], pp. 34, 58–59, 79.

——— 1793. *The Works of Aristotle.* . . . London [no pub.], pp. 27–29, 36, 110, 111, 176, 177.

Armstrong, E. A. 1958. *The Folklore of Birds.* . . . London, Collins, p. 194.

Arnaldus de Villanova. 1494. *Breviarium practicae medicinae* [Venice, Baptista de Tortis], Lib. II, cap. 2.

Aschheim, S. 1930. Die Schwangerschaftsdiagnose aus dem Harne. *Bibl. gynaec. (Basel), 3,* 1–62.

Aschheim, S., and B. Zondek. 1928. Die Schwangerschaftsdiagnose aus dem Harn durch Nachweis des Hypophysenvorderlappenshormons. *Klin. Wschr., 7,* 1404.

Asdell, S. A. 1946. *Patterns of Mammalian Reproduction.* Ithaca, N.Y., Comstock, p. 380.

Ash, John. 1775. *The New and Complete Dictionary of the English Language.* London, E. and C. Dilly.

Atkinson, S. B. 1907. *The Office of Midwife (in England and Wales) under the Midwives Act, 1902 (2 Edw. VII, ch. 17).* . . . London, Baillière, Tindall, and Cox, pp. 2–5, 116.

Augustine, St. 1610. *The City of God.* . . . London, Griffith, Farran, Okeden & Welsh, *1,* Book III, chap. 31.

Avalon, Jean. 1927. Coutumes et pratiques Marocaines dans la grossesse et l'accouchement. *Aesculape,* pp. 138–42.

Aveling, J. H. 1872. *English Midwives; Their History and Prospects.* London, J. & A. Churchill, pp. 1–10, 22–33, 86, 90–91.

—— 1882. *The Chamberlens and the Midwifery Forceps.* . . . London, J. & A. Churchill, pp. 20–24.

Aymar, Alphonse. 1926. Le Sachet accoucheur et ses mystères. . . . *Annales du Midi, 38,* 273–347.

Babcock, W. H. 1888. Folk-tales and folk-lore collected in and near Washington, D.C. *Folk-Lore J., 6,* 85–94.

Baccius, Andreas. 1643. *De gemmis et lapidibus pretiosis.* . . . Francofurti, apud Johannem Davidem Zunnerum, cap. 38, pp. 211–14.

Bacon, Francis. 1676. *Sylva sylvarum.* . . . London, S. G. and B. Griffin, p. 210.

Bächtold-Stäubli, Hanns. 1930–31. *Handwörterbuch des deutschen Aberglaubens.* Berlin and Leipzig, Walter de Gruyter, *3,* 729, 730, 890–91; 1590; *4,* 74, 450.

Bailey, N. 1802. *An Universal Etymological English Dictionary.* Glasgow, Niven, Napier, and Shull.

Baily, Johnson. 1881. [No title] *Notes and Queries,* 6th ser., *3,* 509–10.

Baines, C. C. 1950. Children born with a caul. *Folk-lore, 61,* 104.

Bajerus, J. J. 1708. *Oryctographiae noricae.* . . . Norimbergae, W. Michahellis, pp. 32–33.

Balard, Paul. 1924. Le Contrôle de la profession de sage-femme. *Gaz. hebd. Sci. méd.* Bordeaux, *45,* 6–7.

Bale, John. 1562. *A Newe Comedye or Enterlude / Concernyng Thre Lawes.* . . . London, Thomas Colwell, Act II.

[Ballantyne, J. W.] 1910. The history and etymology of the free-martin. *Brit. med. J., 2,* 1125–26.

Balsamo, Theodorus. 1865. *Canones sanctorum patrum qui in Trullo . . . con-*

venerunt. . . . In: J. P. Migne, *Patrologiae cursus completus.* . . . Paris, *137,* 722–23.

Barb, A. A. 1950. Birds and medical magic. *J. Warburg Courtauld Inst., 13,* 316–22.

Barclay, James. 1799. *A Complete and Universal English Dictionary.* . . . London, G. G. and J. Robinson.

Bargheer, Ernst. 1931. *Eingeweide: Lebens- und Seelenkräfte des Leibesinnern im deutschen Glauben und Brauch.* Berlin and Leipzig, Walter de Gruyter, pp. 155–56.

Baring-Gould, S. 1896. *Curiosities of Olden Times.* Edinburgh, John Grant, p. 62.

Barnes, Henry. 1903. On the bishop's license. *Trans. Cumberland Westmoreland Antiq. Archaeol. Soc.,* n.s., *3,* 59–69.

Barrett, Francis. 1801. *The Magus or Celestial Intelligencer.* . . . London, Lackington, Allen, pp. 10, 39.

Bartelot, R. G. 1923. The eagle stone. *Notes and Queries,* 13th ser., *1,* 113.

Bartels, Max. 1900. Isländischer Brauch und Volksglaube in Bezug auf die Nachkommenschaft. *Z. Ethnol., 32,* 52–86.

Bartels, Paul. 1907. Fortpflanzung, Wochenbett und Taufe in Brauch und Glauben der weissrussischen Landbevölkerung. *Z. Vereins Volksk. Berlin, 17,* 160–71.

Bartholin, Thomas. 1654. *Historiarum anatomicarum rariorum centuria I et II.* Amstelodami, Ioannes Henricus. Historia XCIX.

———— 1673. Ova galli et serpentum. *Acta medica et philosophica hafniensia,* 2, cap. 10.

———— 1676. *Antiquitatum veteris puerperii synopsis.* Amstelodami, Henricus Wetsten, pp. 111–12.

———— 1677. *Neu-verbesserte Kunstliche Zerlegung des Menschlichen Leibes.* Nürnberg, Johann Hoffmann, pp. 321–22.

———— 1684. De ovo praegnante. *Miscellanea curiosa.* . . . Dec. I, 1670, Obs. xxxvi, 104–07.

Bartholomaeus Anglicus. 1539. *Le Propriétaire des choses.* . . . Paris, Nicolas Couteau, *16, 38,* 47.

Bauschius, J. L. 1665. *De lapide aetite schediasma.* . . . Lipsiae, V. J. Trescheri et J.-E. Hahnii, pp. 8–18, 41, 68.

———— 1666. *Anchora sacra, vel scorzonera.* . . . Jenae, J. J. Bauhoferi, p. 160.

Bax, A. R. 1893. Marriage and other licenses in the Commissary Court of Surrey. *Surrey Archaeol. Coll., 11,* 204–43.

Bayle, Pierre. 1741. *A General Dictionary Historical and Critical.* London, James Bettenham, *10,* 356–64.

Bayon, H. P. 1939. Ancient pregnancy tests in the light of contemporary knowledge. *Proc. roy. Soc. B, 32,* 1527–38.

Bayrus, Petrus. 1561. *De medendis humani corporis malis Enchiridion.* . . . Basileae, apud Petrum Pernam, XV, cap. V, pp. 6, 341–42.

B. B. 1852. Derivation of 'caul.' *Notes and Queries,* 1st ser., *5,* 557.

Bechstein, J. M. 1801–09. *Gemeinnützige Naturgeschichte Deutschlands.* Leipzig, *3,* 116 [cited by Butter, 1821].

Beckherus, Daniel. 1660. *Medicus microcosmus.* London, p. 61 [cited by Bourke, 1891].

Beckwith, M. W. 1929. *Black Roadways; A Study of Jamaican Folk Life.* Chapel Hill, University of North Carolina Press, p. 57.

[Beilby, R.] 1791. *A General History of Quadrupeds.* Newcastle upon Tyne, S. Hodgson, R. Beilby, & T. Bewick, p. 33.

Berendes, J. 1902. *Des Pedanios Dioskurides aus Anazarbos Arzneimittellehre.* Stuttgart, F. Enke, *5,* 160, 552.

Bergen, F. D. 1899. *Animal and Plant Lore.* Boston and New York, Houghton, Mifflin, p. 232.

Berthold, A. A. 1849. Transplantation der Hoden. *Arch. Anat. Physiol. wiss. Med., 16,* 42–46.

Best, Henry. 1857. *Rural Economy in Yorkshire in 1641.* . . . Durham, George Andrews, pp. 2, 155, 182.

Bhishagratna, K. K. L. 1907. *An English Translation of the Sushruta Samhita, Based on an Original Sanskrit Text.* Calcutta, K. K. L. Bhishagratna, *1,* xxxiii; *2,* 142.

Bidault, P. 1899. *Les Superstitions médicales du Morvan.* Thèse. Paris, Jouve et Boyer, p. 68.

Bird, Thomas. 1894. An eagle stone. *Notes and Queries,* 8th ser., *5,* 428–29.

Black, W. G. 1883. *Folk-Medicine; A Chapter in the History of Culture.* London, Elliot Stock, pp. 83, 84, 128.

Blackstone, William. 1769. *Commentaries on the Laws of England.* Oxford, Clarendon Press, *4,* vi, 60.

Blake, R. P. 1934. *Epiphanius de gemmis.* . . . London, Christopher's, pp. 117–19.

Blakeborough, Richard. 1898. *Wit, Character, Folklore & Customs of the North Riding of Yorkshire.* London, Henry Frowde, p. 149.

Blakely, S. B. 1937. The diagnosis of the sex of the human fetus in utero. *Amer. J. Obstet. Gynec., 34,* 322–35.

Blencowe, R. W. 1851. Extracts from the parish registers and other parochial documents of East Sussex. *Sussex Archaeol. Coll., 4,* 243–90.

[Blount, Thomas] 1674. *Glossographia; or, A Dictionary Interpreting the Hard Words.* . . . London, Tho. Newcomb.

Blumenbach, [J. F.] 1813. *Commentatio de anomalis et vitiosis quibusdam nisus formativi aberrationibus.* Göttingen, p. 8 [cited by Butter, 1821].

—— 1827. A Manual of Comparative Anatomy. London, W. Simpkin and R. Marshall, p. 361.

Blyth, Edward. 1849. The mammalia, birds, and reptiles. In: Georges Cuvier, ed., *The Animal Kingdom.* London, W. S. Orr, pp. 158–59.

Bodinus, Io. 1581. *De magorum daemonomania.* Basileae, per Thomam Guarinum, Lib. IV, cap. I, p. 317.

[Boemus, Joannes] 1555. *The Fardle of Facions.* . . . London, Iohn Kingstone and Henry Sutton, 2, chap. 11.

Bogdanow, M. 1868. *Biographische Skizze über den Birkhahn,* p. 106 [cited by Brandt, 1889].

Boguet, Henry. 1929. *An Examen of Witches* . . . [London], John Rodker, pp. 69, 88–89.

Bonaciolus, Lud. 1563. *De foetus formatione.* Amstelodami, apud Joannem Ravensteinium, cap. IV, pp. 249–50, 252.

———— 1586. *Enneas muliebris.* Basileae, Conradus Waldkirch, p. 277.

Bonetus, Theophilus. 1686–87. *Medicina septentrionalis.* . . . Geneva, Leonardus Chovët, *1,* 877–88; *2,* 525.

Bonner, Campbell. 1950. *Studies in Magical Amulets, Chiefly Graeco-Egyptian.* Ann Arbor, University of Michigan Press, pp. 79–93.

Bonner, James, and A. W. Galston. 1952. *Principles of Plant Physiology.* San Francisco, W. H. Freeman, p. 355.

Bonser, Wilfrid. 1963. *The Medical Background of Anglo-Saxon England.* . . . London, The Wellcome Historical Medical Library, pp. 265, 269.

[Boorde, Andrew] 1547. *The Breuyary of Helthe.* London, Wyllyam Myddelton, Book II, cap. 71, f. 17.

Boot, A. B. de. 1644. *Le Parfaict Ioaillier, ou histoire des pierreries.* . . . Lyon, Iean-Antoine Hvgvetan, pp. 253, 316, 323, 354, 379, 421, 423–25, 480–86.

Bosworth, Joseph, and T. N. Toller. 1898. *An Anglo-Saxon Dictionary.* . . . Oxford, University Press.

Bouisson, Maurice. 1960. *Magic; Its Rites and History.* London, Rider, p. 148.

Boulart & Chabry. 1882. Sur un Cas d'hermaphrodisme mâle chez l'aigle. *C. R. Soc. Biol. (Paris), 4, 144–45.*

Bourgelat, M. 1769. *Éléments de l'art vétérinaire.* Paris [cited by Thieke, 1911].

Bourgeois, Louise. 1617. *Observations diverses.* . . . Paris, A. Saugrain, p. 206.

Bourke, J. G. 1891. *Scatologic Rites of All Nations.* Washington, D.C., W. H. Lowdermilk, p. 234.

Boyle, Robert. 1672. *An Essay about the Origine and Virtues of Gems.* . . . London, William Godbid, pp. 3, 4.

Boysen Jensen, P. 1936. *Growth Hormones in Plants.* New York and London, McGraw-Hill, p. 67.

Brand, John. 1810. *Observations on Popular Antiquities.* . . . London, Vernon, Hood, and Sharpe, pp. 406–07.

Brandt, Alexander. 1889. Anatomisches und Allgemeines über die sogenannte Hahnenfedrigkeit und über anderweitige Geschlechtsanomalien bei Vögeln. *Z. wiss. Zool., 48,* 101–90.

Braungart, D. C., and R. H. Arnett, Jr. 1962. *An Introduction to Plant Biology.* St. Louis, Mosby, p. 308.

Brinkworth, E. R. C. 1947. Episcopal Visitation Book for the Archdeaconry of Buckingham; 1662. *Buckinghamshire Record Soc., 7,* 4–6, 21–31, 57, 71, 75.

Brissaud, Édouard. 1892. *Histoire des expressions populaires rélatives à l'anatomie, à la physiologie et à la médecine.* Paris, Masson, pp. 320–21.

Brockbank, W. 1958. Mrs. Jane Sharp's advice to midwives. *Med. Hist., 2,* 153–55.

Bromehead, C. N. 1947. Aetites or the eagle-stone. *Antiquity, 21,* 16–22.

Brown, A. R. 1922. *The Andaman Islanders; A Study in Social Anthropology.* Cambridge, University Press, p. 90.

Browne, Thomas. 1646. *Pseudodoxia epidemica.* . . . London, T. H. for Edward Dod, chaps. 2, 7, 22.

Brugsch, Henri. 1863. *Recueil de monuments Egyptiens.* . . . Leipzig, J. C. Hinrichs, *2,* 101–20.

Bruhin, T. A. 1869. Einige ältere Angaben über hahnfedrige Hennen. *Zool. Garten., 10,* 63–64.

Budge, E. A. 1930. *Amulets and Superstitions.* . . . Oxford, University Press, pp. 314–20.

Buffon, G. L. L. 1753. *Histoire naturelle.* Paris, Imprimerie Royale, *4, 214.*

———— 1771. *Histoire naturelle des oiseaux.* Paris, Imprimerie Royale, *2,* 357–58.

Burckhard, Georg. 1911. Einige Dokumente aus dem Anfang des 18. Jahrhunderts zur Hebammenfrage. *Sudhoffs Arch. Gesch. Med., 4,* 129–37.

———— 1912. *Die deutschen Hebammenordnungen von ihren ersten Anfängen bis auf die Neuzeit.* Leipzig, Wilhelm Engelmann, *1,* 26, 29, 49, 99, 100, 104, 109, 123, 131.

Burkhardt Albert. 1941. Untersuchungen über die Wirksamkeit des Oestrons auf Pflanzen bei verschiedener Ernährung. *Ber. Schweiz. Botan. Ges., 51,* 363–94.

Burn, J. S. 1829. *Registrum ecclesiae parochialis.* . . . London, Edward Suter, pp. 81, 84, 85.

Burn, Richard. 1797. *Ecclesiastical Law.* London, A. Strahan, *2,* 513, 515.

Burnet, Gilbert. 1865. *The History of the Reformation.* Oxford, Clarendon Press, *2, 152.*

Burnet, John. 1930. *Early Greek Philosophy.* London, A. and C. Black, pp. 169, 178, 197–98, 244.

Burton, R. F., and L. C. Smithers. 1928. *The Carmina of Caius Valerius Catullus.* New York [no pub.], LXIV, pp. 161, 187.

Buschan, Georg. 1941. *Über Medizinzauber und Heilkunst im Leben der Völker.* . . . Berlin, Oswald Arnold, pp. 548–49.

Butter, John. 1821. An account of the change of plumage exhibited by many species of female birds. . . . *Mem. Wernerian nat. Hist. Soc. (Edinburgh), 3,* 183–206.

Cabanis. 1874. *J. Ornithol., 22,* 344 [cited by Weber, 1890].

Cadiot, P.-J. 1893. *De la Castration du cheval cryptorchide.* Paris, Asselin et Houzeau, pp. 1, 10–11, 14–15.

Candidus Decembrius, Pier. 1498. *De genitura hominis.* . . . [Geneva, L. Cruse, cited by Thorndike, 1934].

Canziani, Estella. 1928. Abruzzese Folklore. *Folk-Lore, 39,* 209–19.

Capivaccius, Hieronymus. 1594. *Practica medicina.* . . . Francofurti, apud Petrum Fischerum, *4, 7,* 9.

Carcopino, Jérôme. 1953. *Etudes d'histoire chrétienne.* . . . Paris, Albin Michel, pp. 12–21, 42–63, 85–91.

Cardanus, Hieronymus. 1554. *De subtilitate.* . . . Basileae, Lvdovicvs Lvcivs, cap. XVIII, p. 500.

———— 1558. *De rerum varietate.* . . . Avinione, per Matthaeum Vincentium, Lib. VIII, cap. xliiii, pp. 427–28.

Cardwell, Edward. 1844. *Documentary Annals of the Reformed Church of England.* . . . Oxford, University Press, pp. 164–65, 203–08, 397–416.

Carič, A. E. 1899. Volksaberglaube in Dalmatien. *Wiss. Mitt. Bosnien Herzegowina (Wien), 6,* 594.

Carlyle, Thomas. 1858. *Translations from the German.* London, Chapman and Hall, p. 362.

Castiglioni, Arturo. 1946. *Adventures of the Mind*. New York, Knopf, pp. 229, 233–35.

Castro, Rodericus à. 1628. *De universa muliebrium morborum medicina*. . . . Hamburgi, Frobbeniano, Lib. III, cap. 7; Lib. IV, cap. 6.

—— 1662. *Medicus politicus*. . . . Hamburgi, Zachariae Hertelii, pp. 153, 216–17.

Celleor, Elizabeth. [1687] *To Dr.* —— *an answer to his queries, concerning the Colledg of Midwives*. London [no pub.], pamphlet.

Cestriensis. 1853. Family caul—child's caul. *Notes and Queries*, 1st ser., 7, 546–47.

Chabas, F. 1862. *La Médecine des anciens Égyptiens*. . . . Chalon-sur-Saone, J. Dejussieu, et Paris, Benjamin Duprat, pp. 68–71.

Chambers, R., ed. 1869. St. Anthony and the pigs: Legal prosecutions of the lower animals. In: *The Book of Days*. London & Edinburgh, W. & R. Chambers, *1*, 126–29.

Chambers, W. J. 1923. The eagle stone. *Notes and Queries*, 12th ser., *12*, 189.

Chanter, H. P. 1923. Folk-lore: Cauls. *Notes and Queries*, 12th ser., *12*, 58.

Chauvaud de Rochefort, C.-J. 1906. *Est-il possible de reconnaître le sexe de l'enfant pendant le cours de la grossesse?* . . . Thèse. Bordeaux, Cadoret, pp. 22, 49.

Chauveau, A. 1873. *The Comparative Anatomy of the Domesticated Animals*. New York, W. R. Jenkins, pp. 897–99.

Chereau, A. 1881. Sorcellerie et magie. In: A. Dechambre, *Dictionaire encyclopédique des sciences médicales*. Paris, G. Masson, *10*, 455–68.

Chesnel, M. A. de. 1856. *Dictionnaire des superstitions, erreurs, préjugés, et traditions populaires*. . . . In: J.-P. Migne, ed. *Troisième encyclopédie théologique*. Paris, Ateliers Catholiques, *20*, col. 109, 738, 1037–40.

Chope, R. P. 1891. The Dialect of Hartland, Devonshire. *English Dialect Soc., 25*, 65.

Chouard, P. 1937. Action combinée de la folliculine et de la durée d'eclairement sur la floraison des reines-marguerites. *C. R. Soc. Biol. (Paris), 126*, 509–12.

Clark, A. J. 1921. Flying ointments. In: M. A. Murray, *The Witch-Cult in Western Europe*. . . . Oxford, Clarendon Press, pp. 279–80.

Clark Hall, J. R., and H. D. Merritt. 1960. *A Concise Anglo-Saxon Dictionary*. Cambridge, University Press.

Clauderus, D. G. 1685. De hippomane. In: *Miscellanea curiosa*. . . . Dec. II, ann. III, obs. lxxiii, pp. 165–66.

Claudinus, I. C. 1607. *Responsionum et consultationum*. . . . Venetiis, apud Hieronymum Tamburinum, Sect. II, cons. 34, pp. 84–85.

Clegg, M. T., J. M. Boda, and H. H. Cole. 1954. The endometrial cups and allantochorionic pouches in the mare with emphasis on the source of equine gonadotrophin. *Endocrinology, 54*, 448–63.

Cobb, J. P. 1883. The diagnosis of the position and sex of the foetus in utero by auscultation. *Clinique (Paris), 4*, 316–17.

Cockayne, Oswald. 1864. *Leechdoms, Wortcunning, and Starcraft of Early England*. . . . London, Longman, *3*, 145.

Cole, L. J. 1927. The lay of the "rooster." *J. Heredity, 18*, 97–106.

Collin de Plancy. 1826. *Dictionnaire infernal*. Paris, P. Mongie, *3*, 249.

Columella, L. J. M. 1745. *Of Husbandry*. London, A. Miller, Lib. VI, caps. 22, 26.

Conklin, G. N. 1958. Alkaloids and the witches' sabbat. *Amer. J. Pharm., 130,* 171–74.

Constantinus Africanus. 1539. De mulierum morbis liber. In: *Opera*. Basileae, apud Henricum Petrum, p. 323.

Copeman, W. S. C. 1960. *Doctors and Disease in Tudor Times*. London, Dawson's, p. 47.

Cortesi, R., C. Tripet, and R. Girard. 1957. Influence de quelques substances hormonales sur le développement et la floraison des bulbes de jacinthes. *Bull. Soc. Pharm. Bordeaux, 96,* 128–32.

Coster, Charles de. 1893. *La Légende et les aventures héroïques, joyeuses, et glorieuses d'Ulenspiegel.* . . . Bruxelles, Paul Lacomblez, p. 1.

Cotta, Iohn. 1612. *A Short Discoverie of the Unobserved Dangers of Severall Sorts of Ignorant and Vnconsiderate* Practisers of Physicke in England. . . . London, William Iones and Richard Boyle, pp. 104, 109–10.

——— 1616. *The Triall of Witch-Craft.* . . . London, George Purslowe, pp. 90, 91.

[Cotton, Charles] 1670. Scarronides: or, Virgile Travestie. . . . London, J. C. for Henry Brome, Book IV, p. 66, lines 15–18.

Courtney, M. A. 1887. Cornish Folk-Lore. *Folk-Lore J., 5,* 177–220.

Craig, Hardin. 1932. *Shakespeare; A Historical and Critical Study.* . . . Chicago, Scott, Foresman, pp. 722–23.

Craigie, W. A. [1931] *A Dictionary of the Older Scottish Tongue.* . . . Chicago, University Press.

Crawley, Ernest. 1902. *The Mystic Rose.* . . . London, Macmillan, pp. 118–19.

Creech [Thomas] 1713. *The Idylliums of Theocritus.* . . . London, E. Cwill, p. 14.

Crisp, Edwards. 1859. Exhibition of a hen that had assumed the plumage of the cock. *Proc. Zool. Soc. London, 27,* 127–28.

Crossley, James. 1845. Potts's Discovery of Witches in the County of Lancaster. . . . *Chetham Soc. Remains Histor. Lit., 6,* 2r.

Cuba, Johannes. c. 1521. *The Noble Lyfe and Natures of Man, of Bestes, Serpentys, Fowles & Fisshes.* [Tran. by L. Andrewe of *Hortus sanitatis*.] Andwarpe, John of Doesborowe, Part I, cap. 125.

Culpeper, Nich. 1653. *A Directory for Midwives.* . . . London, Peter Cole, pp. 101–02.

——— 1700. *A Directory for Midwives.* . . . London [no pub.], pp. 99–100, 107, 110, 111, 292.

——— 1654. *Pharmacopoeia Londinensis.* . . . London, Peter Cole, p. 50.

——— 1672. *The Practice of Physic.* . . . London, p. 505 [cited by Iversen, 1939].

——— 1676. *Culpeper's Last Legacy.* . . . London, J. Phillips, p. 267.

——— 1706. *Riverius reformatus.* . . . London, R. Wellington, p. 338.

Cumming, J. 1870. The stethoscope as a means of diagnosing the sex of the child. *Trans. Edinb. obstet. Soc., 2,* 64–66.

Dalyell, J. G. 1834. *The Darker Superstitions of Scotland.* . . . Edinburgh, Waugh and Innes, pp. 24, 26, 130–32, 134.

Damigeron. 1855. De lapidibus et eorum generibus. In: J. B. Pitra, *Spicilegium solesmense.* . . . Paris, Didot, *3,* 324–35.

Dana, E. S. 1892. *Descriptive Mineralogy.* New York, Wiley.

Darwin, Charles. 1871. *The Descent of Man.* London, John Murray, 2, 180.

Daubenton. 1755. Mémoire sur l'hippomanès. *Hist. Acad. roy. Sci.,* ann. 1751, pp. 293–300.

—— 1756. Observation sur la liqueur de l'allantoïde. *Hist. Acad. roy. Sci.,* ann. 1752, pp. 392–98.

Dawson, W. R. 1929. *Magician and Leech.* . . . London, Methuen, p. 41 et seq.

—— 1934. *A Leechbook or Collection of Medical Recipes of the Fifteenth Century.* . . . London, Macmillan, p. 12.

Dehne, A. 1856. Eine hahnenfedrige Henne. *Allg. dtsch. Naturhist. Z. (Dresden),* n.s., *2,* 67–69.

Delacoux, A. 1834. *Biographie des sages-femmes célébrés.* . . . Paris, Trinquart et L'Auteur, pp. 130–37.

Delaunay. 1921. Les Sages-femmes dans le Maine à la fin de l'ancien régime. *1er Cong. histoire de l'art de guérir, Anvers, 7–12 août 1920,* pp. 283–89.

Delisle. 1902. Vieilles Coutumes et croyances en Languedoc. *Bull. Mém. Soc. Anthrop. (Paris),* 5e sér., *3,* 738–42.

Della Corte, Matteo. 1937 a. Il Crittogramma del "Pater Noster" rinvenuto a Pompei. *Atti della Pont. Acc. Roma di Arch. (ser. 3), Rendiconti. 12,* 397–400.

—— 1937 b. Il Crittogramma del "Pater Noster." *Rendiconti della R. Acc. di Arch., Let. ed Arti Società Reale di Napoli. 12,* 81–99 [cited by Jerphanion, 1938].

Delobson, Dim. 1934. *Les Secrets des sorciers noirs.* Paris, E. Nourry [cited by Klotz, 1947].

Delrio, Martinus. 1608. *Disquisitionum magicarum.* . . . Lugduni, Ioannis Pillehotte, Lib. II, quest. XVI; Lib. III, quest. I, III.

Del Sotto, Is. 1862. *Le Lapidaire du quatorzième siècle.* . . . Vienne, Imprimerie Impériale et Royale, p. 68.

Demič, V. F. 1889. Ueber Volksmedicin in Russland. *Wien. klin. Wschr., 2,* 902–08.

Democritus Junior [Richard Burton]. 1638. *The Anatomy of Melancholy.* Oxford, Henry Cripps, p. 498.

Dennys, N. B. 1876. *The Folklore of China.* . . . London, Trübner, p. 11.

Deveaux. 1743. *L'art de faire des raports en chirurgie.* Paris, d'Houry [cited by Guérin, 1929].

DeVita, Joseph. Personal communication.

Dewhurst, C. J. 1956. Diagnosis of sex before birth. *Lancet, 270,* 471–72.

Dickens, Charles. 1850. *David Copperfield.* London, Bradbury & Evans, p. 1.

Diepgen, Paul. 1937. *Die Frauenheilkunde der alten Welt.* München, J. F. Bergmann, pp. 76–77.

Dinouart, l'Abbé. 1774. *Abrégé de l'embryologie sacrée.* . . . Paris, Nyon, pp. 275–77, 286–87, 291, 494.

Dioscorides, P. A. 1598. *Opera.* . . . [Francofurti], H. A. Wecheli, C. Marnii, et J. Aubrii, pp. 127–28.

Diricq, Ed. 1910. *Maléfices et sortilèges.* . . . Lausanne, Payot, pp. 20, 53–59, 62–63, 78, 100.

Ditton, Martha. [1930] *Die Bedeutung der Frauen bei der Entwicklung der Geburtshilfe.* München, Inaug.-Diss, p. 21.

Domm, L. V., R. G. Gustavson, and Mary Juhn. 1934. Plumage tests in birds. In: Edgar Allen, ed., *Sex and Internal Secretions.* Baltimore, Williams & Wilkins, pp. 608–15.

Drelincurtius, Carolus. 1727. *Opuscula medica.* Hague, apud Gosse & Neaulme, pp. 507–15.

Dryden, John. 1887. *Works.* Edinburgh, William Paterson, *13*, Pastoral IX.

Dugdale, William. 1819. *Monasticon Anglicanum.* . . . London, Longman, Hurst, pp. 184–85.

Durham, M. E. 1909. Some Montenegrin manners and customs. *J. roy. Anthrop. Inst. Great Britain Ireland, 39*, 85–96.

Dwelly, Edward. 1930. *The Illustrated Gaelic Dictionary.* Hants, Edward Dwelly.

Dyer, T. F. F. [1881] *Domestic Folk-Lore.* London, Paris, and New York, Cassell, Petter, Galpin, pp. 3, 4, 125, 126.

Eastman, N. J. 1956. *Williams Obstetrics.* New York, Appleton-Century-Crofts, p. 211.

Eaton, R. J. 1893. The prediction of sex in utero. *Mass. med. J., 13*, 193–96.

Ebers, Georg. 1895. Wie Altägyptisches in die europäische Volksmedicin gelangte. *Z. ägyptische Sprache u. Alterthumskunde, 33*, 1–18.

Edwards, George. 1764. *Gleanings of Natural History.* . . . London, Royal College of Physicians, *3*, chap. 127, p. 168.

Eitel, Martha. 1914. Das bayrische Hebammengewerbe, seine Entwicklung und gegenwärtige Lage. *Ann. ges. Hebammenwesen des In-und Auslandes, 5*, 193–356.

Ekkehard. *Casus Sancti Galli,* cap. 10 [cited by MacKinney, 1937].

Ellin, R. I., and W. J. MacDonald. 1956. An evaluation of the saliva prenatal test . . . *Amer. J. Obstet. Gynec., 72*, 1021–24.

Emanuel, Harry. 1867. *Diamonds and Precious Stones.* . . . London, John Camden, p. 208.

Encelius, Christophorus. 1557. *De re metallica.* . . . Franc[ofurtus], H. C. Egenolphus, pp. 230–34, 243, 314.

Engelmann, G. J. 1884. *Die Geburt bei den Urvölkern.* . . . Wien, Wilhelm Braumüller, p. 12.

Eram, P. 1860. *Quelques Considérations pratiques sur les accouchements en Orient.* Paris, pp. 45, 69, 362 [cited by Ploss et al., 1935].

Erman, A. 1881. Die Sator Arepo Formel. *Z. Ethnol., 13* (suppl.), 35–36.

——— 1887. *Aegypten und Aegyptisches Leben in Altertum.* Tübingen, H. Laupp, *2, 486.*

Eudes-Deslongchamps. 1849–53. Poule éperonné, à plumage de coq. *Mém. Soc. Linnéenne de Normandie, 9,* 21–23.

Evans, E. P. 1906. *The Criminal Prosecution and Capital Punishment of Animals.* New York, Dutton, pp. 162–64.

Evans, Joan. 1922. *Magical Jewels of the Middle Ages and Renaissance.* . . . Oxford, Clarendon Press, pp. 13, 112–20.

———— and M. S. Serjeantson. 1933. *English Mediaeval Lapidaries.* London, Humphrey Milford, pp. 38–57, 119–30.

Fairfax-Blakeborough, J. 1923. Folk-lore: Cauls. *Notes and Queries,* 12th ser., *12,* 9–10.

Farmer, J. S., and W. E. Henley. 1903. *Slang and Its Analogues.* . . . [privately printed, no place], vol. 6.

Fasbender, H. 1897. *Entwickelungslehre, Geburtshilfe und Gynäkologie in den Hippokratischen Schriften.* Stuttgart, Ferdinand Enke, pp. 31–32, 106–07.

Fatio, Victor. 1868. Quelques Observations sur deux Tétras des Musées de Neuchatel et de Lausanne. *Bull. Soc. Vaudoise Sci. nat., 9,* 590–98.

F. C. H. 1857. A child's caul. *Notes and Queries,* 2nd ser., *3,* 397.

Fenning, D. 1775. *The Royal English Dictionary.* . . . London, L. Hawes.

Fenton, E. 1569. *Certaine Secrete Wonders of Nature.* . . . London, Henry Bynneman, p. 41.

Ferckel, Chr. 1912. Zur Gynäkologie und Generationslehre im Fasciculus Medicinae des Johannes de Ketham. *Sudhoffs Arch. Gesch. Med., 6,* 205–22.

Fernie, W. T. 1907. *Precious Stones.* . . . Bristol, John Wright, pp. 341–46.

Ferraris, Lucius. 1746. *Prompta bibliotheca canonica, juridico-moralis theologica.* . . . Venetiis, Franciscum Storti et J. B. Recurti, pp. 445–47.

Festus, S. P., and M. V. Flaccus. 1699. *De verborum significatione.* Amstelodami, Huguet, p. 526.

Fidelis, Fortunatus. 1602. *De relationibus medicorum.* . . . Panormi, apud I. A. de Franciscis, p. 244.

Fleming, George. 1902. *A Text-book of Operative Veterinary Surgery.* New York, W. R. Jenkins, *2,* 584.

Fletcher, Robert. 1896. The witches' pharmacopoeia. *Bull. Johns Hopk. Hosp., 7,* 147–56.

Flügel, D. 1863. *Volksmedizin und Aberglaube im Frankenwalde.* München, pp. 45, 46, 47, 50 [cited by Ploss et al., 1935].

Fontanus, Dionysus. 1560. *De morborum internorum curatione.* Lugduni, Antonium Vincentium, pp. 263–67.

Forbes, T. R. 1949. A. A. Berthold and the first endocrine experiment: Some speculation as to its origin. *Bull. Hist. Med., 23,* 263–67.

———— 1962. William Yarrell, British naturalist. *Proc. Amer. Phil. Soc., 106,* 505–15.

———— 1965. John Hunter on spontaneous intersexuality. *Amer. J. Anat., 116,* 269–300.

Fossel, Victor. 1886. *Volksmedicin und medicinischer Aberglaube in Steiermark.* . . . Graz, Leuschner & Lubensky, pp. 47, 54.

Fossey, C. 1902. *La Magie Assyrienne.* . . . Paris, Ernest Leroux, p. 110.

Franco, P. 1881. Sator-Arepo-Formel. *Z. Ethnol., 30* (suppl.), 333–34.

Frankenhäuser. 1859. Ueber die Herztöne der Frucht und ihre Benutzung zur Diagnose des Lebens, der Stellung, der Lage und des Geschlechts derselben. *Mschr. Geburtsh. Frauenkrankh., 14,* 161–74.

Frazer, J. G. 1919. *Folk-Lore in the Old Testament; Studies in Comparative Religion, Legend and Law.* London, Macmillan, *3*, 441–42.

—— 1935. The magic art and the evolution of kings. In: *The Golden Bough.* New York, Macmillan, *1*, 187–88, 190–91.

Frere, W. H., ed. 1910. *Visitation Articles and Injunctions of the Period of the Reformation,* Vol. III, 1559–75. London, Longmans, Green, 3, 5, 219, 221, 270, 313, 383.

Frere, W. H., and W. M. Kennedy. 1910. *Visitation Articles and Injunctions of the Period of the Reformation.* Vol. II, 1536–1558. London, Longmans, Green, 23, 49, 58–59, 292, 356–57, 360, 372, 385.

Freund, Wilhelm. 1840. *Wörterbuch der lateinischen Sprache.* . . . Leipzig, Hahn, vol. 4.

Friend, J. H., and D. G. Guralnick, eds. 1951. *Webster's New World Dictionary.* . . . Cleveland and New York, World Publishing Co.

Frommann, J. C. 1575. *Tractatus de fascinatione.* . . . Norimbergae, W. M. Endteri & J. A. Endteri, pp. 45–46, 530.

Fühner, Hermann. 1902. *Lithotherapie.* . . . Berlin, S. Calvary, pp. 80, 93–96, 106, 110, 112–13, 118.

Fuller, Thomas. 1719. *Pharmacopoeia extemporanea.* . . . London, W. and J. Innys, pp. 275, 357–58, 419–20.

Galen, Claudius. 1550. *De usu partium corporis humani.* Lugduni, Gulielmum Rouillium, Lib. XV, cap. 4.

Gardner, A. K. 1870. Medical facts and fictions. *Frank Leslie's illus. Newspaper, 30,* 15 Oct., 67.

Gardner, W. U. Personal communication.

Garrison, F. H. 1922. History of endocrine doctrine. In: *Barker's Endocrinology and metabolism.* New York, Appleton, *1,* 45–78.

—— 1929. *An Introduction to the History of Medicine.* . . . Philadelphia and London, Saunders, pp. 150, 237–39, 293.

Gasparri, Petrus. 1933. *Codex iuris canonici.* . . . Vatican. Lib. III, cap. 1, can. 743.

Gemma, Cornelius. 1575. *De naturae divinis characterismis.* . . . Antverpiae, Christophorum Plantinum, Lib. I, cap. 6.

Gentz, Lauritz. 1957. En farmakologisk förklaring av de stora häxprocesserna. *Svensk. Lakartidn., 54,* 2491–2514.

Geoffroy Saint-Hilaire, Isidore. 1822. *Philosophie anatomique.* Paris, pub. by author, *2,* 360–61.

—— 1825. Sur des Femelles de Faisans à plumage de mâles. *Mém. Mus. hist. nat. (Paris), 12,* 220–31.

—— 1841. *Essais de zoologie générale.* . . . Paris, Roret, pp. 493–516.

Georges, K. E. 1880. *Ausführliches lateinisch-deutsches Handwörterbuch.* Leipzig, Hahn.

Gesnerus, Conr. 1586. *Historiae animalium.* . . . Francofurdi, Ioannis Wecheli, *3,* 174–75, 182–84.

Ghalioungui, P., Sh. Khalil, and A. R. Ammar. 1963. On an ancient Egyptian method of diagnosing pregnancy and determining foetal sex. *Med. Hist., 7,* 241–46.

Glück, Leopold. 1894. Die Tatowierung der Haut bei den Katholiken Bosniens und der Herzegowina. *Wiss. Mitt. Bosnien u. Herzegowina (Serajevo)*, 2, 455–62 [cited by Ploss et al., 1935].

Godolphin, John. 1687. *Reportorium canonicum.* . . . London, Christopher Wilkinson, p. 126.

Götz. 1780. Naturgeschichte des Goldphasans. Phasianus pictus Linn. *Naturforsch. 14*, 204–10.

Göz, J. A. 1829. Hans Sachs. . . . Nürnberg, Bauer und Raspe, *1*, 26–30.

Goldie, W. H. 1904. Maori medical lore. *Trans. Proc. New Zealand Inst.*, *37*, 1–120.

Golding, Arthur. 1587. *The Excellent and Pleasant Worke of Iulius Solinus Polyhistor.* . . . London, I. Charlewoode, *13*, 64; *49*, 164.

Goldsmid, Edmund, ed. 1886. *Un-natural History, or Myths of Ancient Science.* . . . Edinburgh, privately printed, *1*, 1–40.

Gollancz, Hermann. 1912. *The Book of Protection.* . . . London, Henry Frowde, p. li.

Goodall, Charles. 1684. *An Historical Account of the College's Proceedings against Empiricks and Unlicensed Practisers, &c.* . . . London, M. Flesher, p. 463.

Googe, Barnabe. 1577. *Fovre Bookes of Husbandry.* . . . London, Richard Watkins, p. 117.

Gordonius, B. 1542. *Omnium aegritudinum à vertice ad calcem.* . . . Parisiis, D. Iacobi, p. 335.

Gosset, Pol. 1909. Les Sages-femmes du pays Rémois au XVIIᵉ et au XVIIIᵉ Siècle. . . . *Union méd. sci. Nord-Est, 33*, 33–39, 43–50, 51–56.

Gove, P. B., ed. 1961. *Webster's Third New International Dictionary.* . . . Springfield, Ill., G. & C. Merriam.

Grant, William, and D. B. Murison. 1956. *The Scottish National Dictionary.* . . . Edinburgh, Scottish Nat. Dictionary Assoc.

Green, Capt. 1836. Note describing a specimen of the Barn-door *Hen* which had assumed the *Cock* plumage. *Proc. Zool Soc. London, 4*, 49.

Greenhill, J. P. 1951. *Principles and Practice of Obstetrics.* Philadelphia and London, Saunders, p. 88.

Gregor, Walter. 1881. *Notes on the Folk-Lore of the North-East of Scotland.* London, Folk-Lore Soc., p. 5.

Grevinus, Jacobus. 1571. *De venenis.* . . . Antverpiae, Christophorum Plantinum, Lib. I, cap. 18.

Grew, Nehemjah. 1681. *Musaeum Regalis Societatis.* . . . London, W. Rawlins, pp. 297–99.

Grgjič-Bjelokosic, Luka. 1899. Volksglaube und Volksbrauch in der Herzegowina. *Wiss. Mitt. Bosnien Herzegowina (Wien)*, 6, 609 [cited by Ploss et al., 1935].

Griffith, F. L. 1898. *The Petrie Papyri.* . . . London, Bernard Quaritch, 2, 9.

—— and Herbert Thompson. 1904. *The Demotic Magical Papyrus of London and Leiden.* London, H. Grevel, col. V, v.

Grillot de Givry. 1929. *Le Musée des sorciers, mages, et alchimistes.* Paris, Librairie de France, p. 58.

Grimm, Jacob. 1883. *Teutonic Mythology.* . . . London, George Bell, 2, 874–75.
—— and Wilhelm Grimm. 1873. *Deutsches Wörterbuch.* Leipzig, S. Hirzel.
Gronovius, Abrahamus. 1768. *Aeliani de natura animalium.* . . . Tubingae, J. G. Cottam, Lib. II, cap. 5, 7; Lib. III, cap. 31.
Grose, Francis. 1811. *A Provincial Glossary.* London, Edward Jeffery, p. 292.
Gross, Johann. 1624. *Kurtze Bassler Chronik.* . . . Basel, Johann Jacob Genath, p. 120.
Grosser, Felix. 1926. Ein neuer Vorschlag zur Deutung der sator-Formel. *Arch. Religionswiss.,* 24, 165–69.
Gruner, O. C. 1930. *A Treatise on the Canon of Medicine of Avicenna.* . . . London, Luzac, pp. 318–19, 347.
Guaccius, F. M. 1626. *Compendium maleficarum.* . . . Mediolani, Ambrosiani, pp. 71, 152–53.
Guainerius, Antonius. 1500. De egritudinibus matricis. In: *Opera medica.* Venetiis, Antonij Moretti per Joannem Hertzog, f. 62–78.
—— 1500. *Practica.* . . . Venetiis [no pub.], cap. 35.
Guarducci, Margherita. 1958. *I graffiti sotto la Confessione di San Pietro in Vaticano.* Città del Vaticano, Libreria Editrice Vaticana, 1, 56.
Guarinonius, Christophorus. 1610. *Consilia medicinalia.* . . . Venetiis, apud Thomam Baglionum, pp. 16–17.
Guérin, F.-P.-M. 1929. *Le Médecin et la justice du XIIIᵉ au XVIIIᵉ siècle en France et en Lorraine.* Thèse. Verdun, H. Fremont, p. 37.
Guillemeau, Charles. 1620. *De la Grossesse et accouchement des femmes.* . . . Paris, Abraham Pacard, p. 15.
Gunther, R. T. 1934. *The Greek Herbal of Dioscorides.* . . . Oxford, University Press, pp. 652, 655–59.
Gurney, J. H. 1888. On the occasional assumption of the male plumage by female birds. *Ibis,* 5th ser., 6, 226–30.
Gurney, J. H., jun. 1886. On a female redstart (*Ruticilla phoenicurus*) assuming the plumage of the male, with remarks on similar instances in other species. *Trans. Norfolk Norwich Nat. Soc.,* 4, 391–92.

Hall, J. R. C. 1931. *A Concise Anglo-Saxon Dictionary.* Cambridge, University Press.
Hallard, J. H. 1894. *The Idylls of Theocritus.* London, Longmans, Green, III, 1–6.
Haller, Albrecht von. 1774. La Génération. . . . Traduite de la Physiologie de M. de Haller. Paris, Des Ventes de la Doué, 2, 23.
—— 1775. *Onomatologia medico-chirurgica completa.* . . . Frankfurt und Leipzig, Stettin, cols. 31, 622.
Halliwell, J. O. 1847. A Dictionary of Archaic and Provincial Words. . . . London, Russell Smith.
Hamilton, Edward. 1860. Exhibition of hen pheasants in male plumage. *Proc. Zool. Soc. London,* 28, 373.
—— 1862. On the assumption of the male plumage by the female of the common pheasant. *Proc. Zool. Soc. London,* 30, 23–25.

Hamlett, G. W. D. 1935. The occurrence of hippomanes within the yolk sac of lemurs. *Anat. Rec., 62,* 279–89.

Hammond, John. 1927. *The Physiology of Reproduction in the Cow.* Cambridge, University Press, p. 161.

Hansemann, D. von. 1914. *Der Aberglaube in der Medizin.* . . . Leipzig, Teubner, pp. 19–20, 27–28.

[Hardouin, Jean] 1714. *Acta conciliorum et epistolae decretales.* . . . Parisiis, ex Typographia Regia, col. 2159.

Harland, John. 1856. The house and farm accounts of the Shuttleworths of Gawthorpe Hall . . . from September 1582 to October 1621. *Chetham Soc., Remains Histor. Lit., 35,* 189, 198.

———, ed. 1864. A volume of Court Leet records of the Manor of Manchester in the sixteenth century. *Chetham Soc., Remains Histor. Lit., 63,* 30.

Hartland, E. S. 1890. Fairy births and human midwives. *Archaeol. Rev. (London), 4,* 328–43.

Hartshorne, Albert. 1909. Notes on lodestones and eagle stones. *Proc. Soc. Antiquaries (London),* 2nd ser., *22,* 512–18.

Harvey, William. 1653. *Anatomical Exercitations.* . . . London, James Young for Octavian Pulleyn, Exercit. XIII.

Hastings, James, ed. 1910, 1911, 1919. *Encyclopaedia of Religion and Ethics.* New York, Scribner's *2,* 635, 639, 663; *3,* 358, 359, 361, 394; *8,* 44–45; *10,* 242–43.

Haverfield F. 1899. A Roman charm from Cirencester. *Archaeol. J., 56,* 319–23.

Hazlitt, W. C., ed. 1870. *Popular Antiquities of Great Britain.* . . . London, John Russell Smith, pp. 139–42.

——— 1905. *Faiths and Folklore; A Dictionary.* . . . London, Reeves and Turner, *1,* 99–101.

Heim, Ricardus. 1893. Incantamenta magica graeca latina. *Jahrb. class. Philologie von A. Fleckeisen., 19* (suppl.), 463–576.

Heinsius, Theodor. 1820. *Volksthümliches Wörterbuch der deutschen Sprache.* . . . Hannover, Hahn, vol. 3.

Henderson, William. 1866. *Notes on the Folk Lore of the Northern Counties of England and the Borders.* London, Longmans, Green, pp. 14, 43.

Hendrie, Robert, trans. 1847. *An Essay upon Various Arts in Three Books by Theophilus.* . . . London, John Murray, Lib. III, cap. 48.

Henriksen, Erle. 1941. Pregnancy tests of the past and present. *Western J. Surg. Obstet. Gynec., 49,* 567–75.

Herlicium, D. D. 1628. *De curationibus gravidarum, puerparum, et infantum.* . . . Alte Stettin, David Rheren, pp. 253–71.

Herold, Ludwig. 1953. Volksbrauch und Volksglaube bei Geburt und Taufe im Karlsbader Bezirk. *Hess. Blätt. Volkskunde, 44,* 5–49.

Herrgott, F.-J. 1895. *Soranus d'Éphese . . . et Moschion.* . . . Nancy, Berger-Levrault, pp. 42–44.

Hervé, G. 1906. De Charles Estienne et de quelques recettes et superstitions médicales au XVIe siècle. *Rev. École d'Anthrop. Paris, 16,* 133–39.

Heyse, J. C. A. 1842. *Handwörterbuch der deutschen Sprache.* . . . Magdeburg, Wilhelm Heinrichshofen.

Hildegardis, Sancta. 1855. Opera omnia. In: *Patrologiae cursus completus.* . . .
Ed. by J.-P. Migne, Paris, [no pub.], *197,* col. 1257.

Hilton-Simpson, M. W. 1922. Arab Medicine and Surgery. . . . London, Oxford
University Press, p. 89.

Hiltprandus, Joannes. 1595. *Ordnung und nutzliche Vnderweysung für die
Hebammen vnd Schwangeren Frawen.* . . . Passaw, M. Henninger [cited
by Klein, 1910].

Hirschfeld, Otto, ed. 1888. *Inscriptiones Galliae Narbonensis latinae.* . . . Berolini
apud Georgium Reimerum, p. 20.

Hobday, F. T. G. 1903. *The Castration of Cryptorchid Horses and the Ovariot-
omy of Troublesome Mares.* Edinburgh and London, W. & A. K. Johnston,
pp. 17, 36, 47–49.

Höfler, M. 1893. *Volksmedizin und Aberglaube in Oberbayerns Gegenwart und
Vergangenheit.* München, Otto Galler, pp. 39, 199–200.

Hoffman, Walther. 1934. Versuche zur Schwangerschaftsdiagnose aus dem Harn.
Dtsch. med. Wschr., 60, 822–24.

Hole, Christina. 1957. Notes on some Folklore Survivals in English Domestic
Life. *Folk-Lore, 68,* 411–19.

Holthausen, F. 1897. Rezepte, Segen und Zauberspruche aus zwei Stockholmer
Handschriften. *Anglia, 19,* 75–88.

—— 1934. *Altenglisches etymologisches Wörterbuch.* Heidelberg, Carl Winter.

Holzinger, J. B. 1883. *Zur Naturgeschichte der Hexen.* Graz, Naturwiss. Verein
f. Steiermark, pp. 14–15.

Home, Everard. 1799. An account of the dissection of a hermaphrodite dog. To
which are prefixed, some observations on hermaphrodites in general. *Phil.
Trans. roy. Soc. B, 1,* 157–78.

—— 1823. On animals imperfectly or preternaturally formed at the time of
their birth. In: *Lectures on Comparative Anatomy.* London, Longmans,
3, 329–30.

Homeyer, Alexander von. 1868. Hahnfedrig oder gehörnt und doch fruchtbar.
Zool. Garten., 9, 94–97.

Hood, Thomas. 1857. The sea-spell. In: *The poetical works of Thomas Hood.* . . .
Boston, Phillips, Sampson.

Hopf, Ludwig. 1888. *Thierorakel und Orakelthiere in alter und neuer Zeit.* . . .
Stuttgart, Kohlhammer, pp. 164–65.

Hovorka, Oskar von. 1915. *Geist der Medizin.* . . . Wien und Leipzig, Wilhelm
Bräumuller, p. 235.

—— and A. Kronfeld. 1908–09. *Vergleichende Volksmedizin.* . . . Stuttgart,
Strecker & Schröder, *1,* 8, 25, 188; *2,* 327, 525–27, 528–34, 564, 593–
94.

Hoy, J. D. 1831. Observations on the British species of shrikes, their habits, nid-
ification, &c. *Loudon's Mag. nat. Hist., 4,* 341–44.

Hucherus, Ioannis. 1610. *De sterilitate utriusque sexus.* . . . Coloniae Allobro-
gum, apud Samuelem Crispinum, pp. 582–84.

Hughes, Pennethorne. 1952. *Witchcraft.* London, Longmans, Green, pp. 59, 70.

Hull, Eleanor. 1928. *Folklore of the British Isles.* London, Methuen, pp. 76, 187,
192, 193.

Hunter, John. 1779. Account of the free martin. *Phil. Trans. roy. Soc. B, 69,* 279–93.

——— 1780. Account of an extraordinary pheasant. *Phil. Trans. roy. Soc. B, 70,* 527–35.

——— 1792. A description of the situation of the testis in the foetus, with its descent into the scrotum. In: *Observations on Certain Parts of the Animal Oeconomy.* London. G. Nicol and J. Johnson, p. 18.

Hunter, Robert, and Charles Morris. 1897. *Universal Dictionary of the English Language.* . . . New York, P. F. Collier.

Hurd-Mead, K. C. 1938. *A History of Women in Medicine.* Haddam, Conn., Haddam Press, pp. 313, 521, 523.

Hutchinson, G. E. 1955. The Enchanted Voyage: A Study of the Effects of the Ocean on Some Aspects of Human Culture. *Sears Found.: J. Marine Res., 14,* 276–83.

H. W. R. 1894. An eagle stone. *Notes and Queries,* 8th ser., *5,* 518.

Hyde, W. W. 1916. The prosecution and punishment of animals and lifeless things in the Middle Ages and modern times. *U. Penna. Law Rev., 64,* 696–730.

Hyrtl, Joseph. 1884. *Die alten deutschen Kunstworte der Anatomie.* Wien, Wilhelm Bräumuller, pp. 81–82.

Isidorus. [1493] *Ethimologiarum* [no place, no pub.], Lib. XVI, cap. 4.

Iversen, Erik. 1939. Papyrus Carlsberg No. VII, With Some Remarks on the Egyptian Origin of Some Popular Birth Prognoses. København, Ejnar Munksgaard, pp. 1–31.

Jacobs, Julius. 1894. *Het Familie- en Kampongleven op Groot-Atjeh.* Leiden [cited by Ploss et al., 1935].

Jahn, Ulrich. 1886. Hexenwesen und Zauberei in Pommern. *17. Kong. Dtsch. Anthrop. Ges. in Stettin* [cited by Ploss et al., 1935].

James, F. 1956. Sexing foetuses by examination of amniotic fluid. *Lancet, 270,* 202–03.

James, R. 1743. A Medicinal Dictionary. . . . London, T. Osborne, vol. 1.

Jamieson, John. 1882. *An Etymological Dictionary of the Scottish Language.* . . . Paisley, Alexander Gardner, vol. 4.

Jenner, Edward. 1931. *The Note-Book of Edward Jenner.* . . . Oxford, University Press, p. 28.

Jerphanion, G. de. 1938. (1) La Formule magique: *'Sator Arepo'* ou *'rotas opera';* vieilles théories et faits nouveaux. (2) À propos des Exemplaires, trouvés à Pompei, du carré magique *'Rotas Opera.'* (3) Une nouvelle Hypothèse sur l'origine du carré magique. In: *La Voix des monuments.* Rome et Paris, Études d'Archéologie, pp. 38–76, 77–89, 90–94.

Johannes Anglicus de Gatisden. 1492. *Rosa anglica practica medicinae a capite ad pedes.* Pavia, L. Gerta for J. A. Birretta, ff. 104 v., 105 r.

Johanneson, Alexander. 1956. *Isländisches etymologisches Wörterbuch.* Bern, Francke.

Johnson, Samuel. 1805. *A Dictionary of the English Language.* . . . London, Longman, Hurst, Rees, and Orme, vol. 3.

Johnson, Tho., trans. 1665. *The Workes of that Famous Chirurgion Ambrose Parey.* . . . London, E. C., Book XXI, chap. 19.

Jones, William. 1880. *Credulities Past and Present.* . . . London, Chatto and Windus, pp. 111, 367, 388, 449, 462.

Jonson, Ben. 1903. *The Alchemist.* . . . London, De La Mare, *I*, 1, 327.

Joubert, Laur. 1578. *Erreurs populaires.* . . . Bourdeaus, S. Millanges, Liv. III, chap. 3; Liv. IV, chap. 6.

J. T. F. 1899. A child's caul. *Notes and Queries,* 9th ser., *3*, 26.

———— 1904. *Notes and Queries,* 10th ser., *1*, 26.

Juvenalis, D. J. 1928. *Satires.* . . . London, Heinemann, VI, 614–17.

Kanner, Leo. 1931. Born with a caul. *Med. Life, 38*, 528–48.

Karusis, Antonio. 1913. Pregiudizi popolari Putignanesi (Bari). *Arch. Antropol. Etnol. (Firenze), 17*, 311–32.

Kaufmann, Raphaël. 1906. *Pratiques et superstitions médicales en Poitou.* Thèse, Paris, p. 66.

Kaumann, Franz. 1906. Der Adlerstein als Hülfsmittel bei der Geburt. *Hess. Blätt. Volkskunde (Leipzig), 5*, 133–56.

Kemp, P. 1935. *Healing Ritual.* . . . London, Faber and Faber, pp. 125–26.

Kern, Hans. 1929. *Zur Geschichte des Hebammenwesens in Basel.* Inaug.-Diss. Basel, Emil Birkhäuser, p. 34.

Kershasp, P. 1904. Some superstitions prevailing amongst the Canarese-speaking people of Southern India. *J. anthrop. Soc. Bombay, 7*, 83–88.

Kerslake, Thomas. 1850. Midwives licensed. *Notes and Queries,* 1st ser., *2*, 499.

Kéténedjian, H. 1918. Les pratiques obstétricales en Arménie (superstition, magie, sorcellerie et fétichisme). Thèse, Paris, Le François, p. 22 et seq.

Khunrath, Conradus. 1623. *Medulla destillatoria.* . . . Hamburg, Frobenianum, p. 102.

King, C. W. 1865. *The Natural History, Ancient and Modern, of Precious Stones and Gems and of the Precious Metals.* London, Bell and Daldy, pp. 49–50.

Kinloch, G. R. 1848. *Reliquiae antiquae Scoticae.* . . . Edinburgh, T. G. Stevenson, pp. 20, 113, 114, 121.

Kircherus, Athanasius. 1665. *Arithmologia.* . . . Romae, Varesij, pp. 64, 220.

Kittredge, G. L. 1929. *Witchcraft in Old and New England.* Cambridge, Harvard University Press, pp. 114–15.

Klein, G. 1902. Ueber Hebammenbücher aus 1½ Jahrtausenden. *Bayer. Hebammen-Z.,* pp. 3–13.

Klotz, Pierre. 1947. *Le Diagnostic du sexe foetal durant la grossesse.* Paris, G. Doin.

Knortz, Karl. 1909. *Der menschliche Körper in Sage, Brauch und Sprichwort.* Würzburg, Curt Kabitsch, p. 21.

Kögl, Fritz, A. J. Haagen-Smit, and Hanni Erxleben. 1933a. Studien über das Vorkommen von Auxinen im menschlichen und im tierischen Organismus. 7. Mitteilung über pflanzliche Wachstumsstoffe. *Hoppe-Seyler's Z. physiol. Chem., 220*, 137–61.

———— 1933b. Über ein Phytohormon der Zellstreckung. Reindarstellung des Auxins aus menschlichen Harn. 4. Mitteilung über pflanzliche Wachtumsstoffe. *Hoppe-Seyler's Z. physiol. Chem., 214*, 241–61.

Köhler, Reinhold. 1881. Sator-Arepo-Formel, *Z. Ethnol., 30* (suppl.), 301–06.

Koenig-Warthausen. 1854. *Naumannia,* p. 34 [cited by Stölker, 1875].

Korschelt, E. 1888. Sur un Cas de 'plumage de mâle' chez une Cane domestique. *Bull. biol. France Belgique, 19,* 110–13.

Kräutermann, Valentino. 1730. *Der Thuringische Theophrastus Paracelsus Wunder- und Kräuterdoctor.* Arnstadt und Leipzig, Ludwig Niedt, pp. 254–57.

Krauss, H. 1913. Zur Geschichte des Hebammenwesens im Fürstentum Ansbach. *Arch. Gesch. Med., 6,* 64–71.

Krauss, Samuel. 1911. *Talmudische Archäologie, 2,* 3–4.

Kühn, C. G., ed. 1827. Claudius Galen. De remediis parabilibus, Lib. 2, cap. XXVI. In: *Medicorum Graecorum opera quae exstant.* Lipsiae, Car. Cnoblochii, Lib. XIV, p. 476.

Kunz, G. F. 1915. *The Magic of Jewels and Charms.* Philadelphia and London, Lippincott, pp. 67, 131, 151–52, 173, 177–78.

Kurath, Hans, and S. M. Kuhn. 1959. *Middle English Dictionary.* Ann Arbor, University of Michigan Press.

La Brousse, de, et al. 1771. Observations sur la connaissance du pouls dans les grossesses, qui peut servir à distinguer les mâles & les femelles, avant l'accouchement. . . . *J. méd. chir. pharm. (Paris), 36,* 121–29, 129–41.

Lachs, Johann. 1903. *Die Gynaekologie des Galen.* . . . Breslau, J. U. Kern, p. 32.

Lacroix, J. V. 1949. Orchiectomy (Castration). In: H. P. Hoskins and J. V. Lacroix, eds. *Canine Surgery.* . . . Evanston, Ill., *North American Veterinarian,* pp. 401–02.

Lalung, H. de. 1939. *L'Accouchement à travers les âges et les peuples.* Paris, Cortial, p. 25.

Lammert, G. 1869. *Volksmedizin und medizinischer Aberglaube in Bayern.* . . . Würzburg, F. A. Julien, pp. 158, 160, 169.

Lapeyronie. 1710. Observation sur les petits oeufs de poule sans jaune, que l'on appelle vulgairement oeuf de coq. *Hist. Acad. roy. Sci.,* pp. 553–60.

Larcher, O. 1873. Mémoire sur les affections des parties génitales femelles chez les oiseaux. *J. Anat. (Paris), 9,* 565–85.

Last, Hugh. 1954. Jérôme Carcopino: Études d'histoire Chrétienne. Le Christianisme secret du carré magique: Les fouilles de Saint-Pierre et la tradition. . . . *J. Roman Stud., 44,* 112–16.

Lavrembergvs, Gvilelmus. 1627. *Historica descriptio aetitis seu lapidis aquilae* . . . Rostochi, A. Ferberi.

Lea, H. C. 1939. *Materials Toward a History of Witchcraft.* Philadelphia, University of Pennsylvania Press, *1,* 276–85, 292–95, 358–65; *2,* 670–89.

Leach, Maria, ed. 1949. *Funk & Wagnalls' Standard Dictionary of Folklore, Mythology and Legend.* New York, Funk & Wagnalls.

Lean, V. S. 1903. *Lean's Collectanea.* Bristol, J. W. Arrowsmith, *2,* 99.

Le Boursier du Coudray, A. M. 1777. *Abrégé de l'art des accouchements.* . . . Paris, Debure, p. 7.

[LeBrun, P., and J. B. Thiers] 1733–36. *Superstitions anciennes et modernes: Préjugés vulgaires.* . . . Amsterdam, J. F. Bernard, *1,* 77; *2,* 16.

Lefèvre, L.-R. 1948. *Journal de L'Estoile pour le regne de Henri IV.* Paris, Gallimard, *1, 21* Oct. 1596.

Lemnius, Laevinus. 1658. *The Secret Miracles of Nature.* . . . London, Jo. Streater, pp. 105, 270–71; Book VII.

Leonardus, Camillus. 1750. *The Mirror of Stones.* . . . London, J. Freeman, pp. 76–77, 99–100, 101, 102, 105, 107–08, 112–13, 206–10, 215, 219, 230.

Leuckart, R. 1853. Zeugung. In: Rudolph Wagner. *Handwörterbuch der Physiologie.* Braunschweig, F. Vieweg, *4,* 753.

Levaillant, François. 1706. *Histoire naturelle des oiseaux d'Afrique.* Paris, Delachaussée, *5,* 42.

Levret, André. 1766. *Essai sur l'abus des regles générales, et contre les préjugés qui s'opposent aux progrès de l'art des accouchemens.* Paris, Prault, Didot, pp. 52, 93–96.

Lewis, C. T., and Charles Short, eds. 1907. *A New Latin Dictionary.* New York, American Book.

Lillie, F. R. 1917. The free-martin; A study of the action of sex hormones in the foetal life of cattle. *J. exp. Zool., 23,* 371–452.

Lin, Ta-Jung, Alois Vasicka, and A. E. Bennett. 1960. Prenatal determination of the sex of the baby. *Amer. J. Obstet. Gynec., 79,* 938–42.

Lind, L. R., trans. 1963. *Aldrovandi on Chickens.* . . . Norman, University of Oklahoma Press, p. 60.

Littré, E., ed. 1844. *Oeuvres complètes d'Hippocrate.* . . . Paris, J.-B. Baillière, *5,* 137; *6,* 501; *7,* 417, 511; *8,* 415, 417, 486.

———— 1850. *Histoire naturelle de Pline.* . . . Paris, Dubochet, Le Chevalier, *7, 5; 10,* 4; *30,* 44; *36,* 39, 40; *37,* 59, 66.

Livius, Titus. 1919. *Ab urbe condita.* Trans. B. O. Foster. London, Heinemann, Book XXII, line 13.

Lonicerus, Adamus. 1560. *Kreuterbüch.* . . . Franckfort am Meyn, Christian Egenolff, ff. 29, 35, 58, 59.

Lorenz, Th. 1887. *Beitrag zur Kenntnis der ornithol. Fauna an der Nordseite des Kaukasus,* Moscow, p. 57 [cited by Brandt, 1889].

Lovell, Robert. 1661. Παυζωορυκτολογια, *sive panzoologico-mineralogia, or A Compleat History of Animals and Minerals.* . . . Oxford, Hen. Hall, pp. 73, 74, 76, 83, 85, 87, 89, 91, 94, 246.

Lovett Edward. 1925. *Magic in Modern London.* Croydon, *Advertizer* Offices, pp. 52–53.

Lucanus, M. A. 1928. *De bello civili.* London, Heinemann, Lib. VI, pp. 454–56, 670–76.

Lüring, H. E. L. 1888. *Die über die medicinischen Kenntnisse der alten Ägypter berichtenden Papyri vergleichen mit den medicinischen Schriften griechischer römischer Autoren.* Inaug.-Diss. Leipzig, Breitkopf & Härtel, pp. 4, 5, 135–41.

Lush, J. L., J. M. Jones, and W. H. Dameron. 1930. The Inheritance of Cryptorchidism in Goats. *Texas Agric. exp. Sta. Bull.,* no. 7, Feb.

MacCulloch, J. A., ed. 1930. *The Mythology of All Races.* Boston, Marshall Jones, *2,* 235.

MacDonald, A. D. 1883. The antegenetic discovery of foetal sex. *Lancet, 1,* 222.

Macht, D. I. 1946. Influence of estrone, progesterone, and stilbestrol on growth of Lupinus seedlings. *Med. Rec. (N.Y.), 159,* 164–66.

Mackenzie, George. 1678. The Laws and Customes of Scotland. . . . Edinburgh, George Swintoun, pp. 81–108.

MacKinney, L. C. 1937. *Early Mediaeval Medicine with Special Reference to France and Chartres.* Baltimore, Johns Hopkins Press, p. 45.

Macleod, Norman, and Daniel Dewar. 1845. *A Dictionary of the Gaelic Language.* London, Bohn.

MacMichael, J. H. 1905. Palindrome. *Notes and Queries,* 10th ser., *3,* 310.

Männling, J. C. 1713. *Denckwürdige Curiositäten.* . . . Franckfurth und Leipzig, Michael Rohrlach, p. 174.

Magie, David, trans. 1924. *The Scriptores historiae Augustae.* London, Heinemann, II, 4.

Makowski, E. L., K. A. Prem, and I. H. Kaiser. 1956. Detection of sex of fetuses by the incidence of sex chromatin body in nuclei of cells in amniotic fluid. *Science, 123,* 542–43.

Malgaigne, J.-F. 1840. *Oeuvres complètes d'Ambroise Paré.* . . . Paris, J.-B. Baillière, Liv. 18, chaps. 5, 12.

Malins, E. 1874–75. Note on obstetric superstition. *Obst. J. Great Britain Ireland, 2,* 9–10.

Manchester, H. L. 1887. Predicting the sex of the unborn. *Med. surg. Reporter (Philadelphia), 57,* 61.

Manger, Julius. 1933. Untersuchungen zum Problem der Geschlechtsdiagnose aus Schwangerenharn. *Dtsch. med. Wschr., 59,* 885–87.

[Mannyng, Robert] 1862. *Roberd of Brunne's Handlyng Synne (written A.D. 1303).* . . . London, J. B. Nichols, pp. 297–98, 9592–9649.

Marbodeus. 1740. *De lapidibus pretiosis enchiridion.* . . . [No place] Bruckmann, pp. 41–43, 58.

Marcus, J. H. 1917. Childbirth and its ancient customs. *N. Y. med. J., 106,* 1213–16.

Marine, David. 1935. The physiology and principal interrelations of the thyroid. In: *Glandular Physiology and Therapy* . . . Chicago, Amer. Med. Assoc., p. 326.

Markham, Geruase. 1607. Cavelarice; or the English Horseman. . . . London, Edward White, *1,* 50.

Marqués-Rivière, Jean. 1950. *Amulettes, talismans et pantacles dans les traditions orientales et occidentales.* Paris, Payot, p. 168.

Marshall, Mark. 1948. The kyesteine pellicle; An early biological test for pregnancy. *Bull. Hist. Med., 22,* 178–95.

Marshall, W. H. 1873. *Provincialisms of East Yorkshire; by Mr Marshall; 1788.* London, Trübner, p. 35.

Martin, M. 1934. *A description of the Western Islands of Scotland circa 1695.* . . . Stirling, Eneas Mackay, pp. 176–77.

Martius, C. F. P. von. 1867. *Zur Ethnographie Amerika's zumal Brasiliens.* Leipzig, Friedrich Fleischer, *1,* 731–32.

Martius, J. N. 1719. *Unterricht von der wunderbaren Magie und derselben med-*

icinischen Gebrauch. . . . Frankfurth und Leipzig, C. G. Nicolai, pp. 121–23.

Marzell, Heinrich. 1963. *Zauberpflanzen-Hexentränke; Brauchtum und Aberglaube.* Stuttgart, Franck, pp. 47–48.

Mason-Hohl, Elizabeth, trans. 1940. *The Diseases of Women, by Trotula of Salerno.* . . . Los Angeles, Ward Ritchie, pp. vii, 18; chaps. 16, 17.

Massaria, Alexandrus. 1601. *Practica medica.* . . . Francofurti, Melchioris Hartmanni, *11,* 587; *12,* 591.

Matignon, J. J. 1895. Comment les Chinois prétendent durant la vie intra-utérine, arriver à reconnaître le sexe du foetus. *Arch. tocol. gynéc.,* 22, 406–09.

Mattei. 1876. Note sur les pulsations cardiaques du foetus, indiquant par leur fréquence le sexe de l'enfant pendant la grossesse. *Arch. tocol. gynéc., 3,* 167–68.

Maugray, John. 1724. *The Female Physician.* . . . London, James Holland, p. 73.

Mauduy. 1849. Observations sur les changements qui s'opèrent dans le plumage des oiseaux, soit par l'âge, ou tout autre cause. *Actes Soc. Linn. Bordeaux, xxx 16,* 304–06.

Maurer, Konrad. 1860. *Isländische Volkssagen der Gegenwart.* . . . Leipzig, J. C. Hinrich, pp. 180–81.

Mauriceau, François. 1675. *Traité des maladies des femmes grosses.* . . . Paris, chez l'Auteur, pp. 97–100.

—— 1755. *The Diseases of Women with Child and Child-Bed.* . . . London, R. Ware, p. 132.

McGavack, T. H. 1951. *The Thyroid.* St. Louis, Mosby, p. 218.

McKee, E. S. 1886. The early diagnosis of pregnancy. *J. Amer. med. Ass. 7,* 510–12.

McKenzie, Dan. 1927. *The Infancy of Medicine.* London, Macmillan, pp. 305, 327.

Meckel, J. F. 1824. *System der vergleichende Anatomie.* Halle, vol. 1 [cited by Brandt, 1889].

M. E. F. 1850. Boy or girl. *Notes and Queries,* 1st ser., 2, 20.

Mercurio, Scipion. 1621. *La commare o riccoglitrice.* Venetia, Ciotti, *1,* 57.

Meyer, R. 1866. Ein Haushuhn mit Hahnengefieder. *Zool. Garten., 7,* 167–70.

M. G. W. P. 1897. The caul, silly-how, or silly-hood. *Notes and Queries,* 8th ser., *11,* 234.

Middleton, Thomas. 1950. *The Witch.* Oxford, University Press, I, 2; V, 3.

Migne, L'Abbé. 1856. Encyclopédie théologique. Paris, J.-P. Migne. 20 cols. 225–26.

Miller, W. C., and G. P. West. 1953. *Black's Veterinary Dictionary.* London, Adam and Charles Black.

Mizaldus, Antonius. 1719. *Hundert nützliche curieuse und angenehme Kunst-Stücke.* Frankfurth und Leipzig, C. G. Nicolai, p. 325.

M. N. 1900. Installation of a midwife. *Notes and Queries,* 9th ser., 6, 274.

Mommsen, Th., ed. 1864. *C. lvlii Solini: Collectanea rerum memorabilium.* Berolini, Friderici Nicolai, pp. 141–42.

Moore, A. W. 1891. *The Folk-Lore of the Isle of Man.* . . . London, D. Nutt, p. 157.

Moorehouse, G. W. 1898. Bits of medical folk-lore. *Boston med. surg. J., 138,* 201–02.

Moss, L. W., and S. C. Cappanari. 1960. Folklore and medicine in an Italian village. *J. Amer. Folklore, 73,* 95–102.

M. P. 1889. Folk-lore: Caul. *Notes and Queries,* 7th ser., *8,* 284.

Muralt, Johann von. 1697. *Kinder- und Hebammen-Buchlein.* Zürich, E. & J. König, pp. 53–54.

Murray, J. A. H. 1893–1901. *A New English Dictionary on Historical Principles.* . . . Oxford, Clarendon Press.

Murray, M. A. 1918. Child-sacrifice among European witches. *Man, 18,* 60–62.

—— 1921. *The Witch-Cult in Western Europe.* . . . Oxford, Clarendon Press, pp. 279–80.

—— 1937. Witchcraft. In: *The Encyclopaedia Britannica.* London, Encyclopaedia Britannica, *23,* 686–88.

Myrc, John. 1868. *Instructions for Parish Priests.* London, Trübner, lines 87–102.

Naumann, J. A. 1846–53. *Naturgeschichte der Vögel Deutschlands.* . . . Stuttgart, vol. 13 [cited by Brandt, 1889].

Neilson, W. A., ed. 1944. *Webster's New International Dictionary of the English Language.* Springfield, Mass., G. & C. Murray.

Neuburger, Max. 1910. *History of Medicine.* London, Oxford University Press, *1,* 59, 63.

Nevinson, Charles, ed. 1852. *Later Writings of Bishop Hooper.* . . . Cambridge, University Press, pp. 140–41.

Newman, Barbara, and Leslie Newman. 1939. Some birth customs in East Anglia. *Folk-Lore, 50,* 176–87.

Nicholson, John. 1890. *Folk Lore of East Yorkshire.* London, Simpkin, Marshall, Hamilton, Kent, p. 1.

Nicholson, William, ed. 1843. *The Remains of Edmund Grindal, D.D.* . . . Cambridge, University Press, pp. 156–57, 174.

Nicols, Thomas. 1653. *Arcula gemmea.* . . . London, Nath. Brooke, pp. 134, 184–89, 200.

Nilsson, S. 1845. Ueber Auer-, Birk- und Pfau-Hennen und weibliche Enten mit männlichem Gefieder, so wie über Bastarde von Auer-, Birk- und Schnee-Hühnern. *Arch. skand. Beitr. Naturgesch., 1,* 397–412.

Nonius Marcellus. 1895. *De conpendiosa doctrina.* Oxford, Clarendon Press, p. 206.

Norman, H. J. 1933. Witch ointments. Appendix to: Montague Summers, *The Werewolf.* London, Kegan Paul, Trench, Trübner, p. 291.

Notestein, Wallace. 1911. *A History of Witchcraft in England from 1558 to 1718.* Washington, D.C., Am. Hist. Assoc., pp. 20–21, 41, 258–59.

O'Connor, J. J. 1931. *Dollar's Veterinary Surgery.* Chicago, Alex. Eger, pp. 333, 671–73.

Oefele. 1899. Jaspis als Geburtsamulet. *Allg. med. Central-Ztg.,* pp. 224–25.

Oldys, William. 1809. *The Harleian Miscellany.* . . . London, White, p. 142.

O'Malley, C. D. 1964. *Andreas Vesalius of Brussels, 1514–1564.* Berkeley and Los Angeles, University of California Press, p. 28.

—— and J. B. deC. M. Saunders. 1952. *Leonardo da Vinci on the Human Body.* . . . New York, Henry Schuman, p. 470.

Ovidius Naso, P. 1947. *Amores.* Cambridge, Harvard University Press, I, 8.

Owen, H., and J. B. Blakeway. 1825. *A History of Shrewsbury.* London, Harding, Lepard, 2, 362–64.

Pachinger, A. M. 1904. Der Aberglaube vor und bei der Geburt des Menschen. *Muench. med. Wschr., 51,* 1438–39.

—— 1906. Die Geburt in Glauben und Brauch der Deutschen in Oberöster-reich, Salzburg und den Grenzgebieten. *Anthropophyteia, 3,* 34–40.

Palmer, A. S. 1883. *Folk-Lore Etymology.* . . . New York, Henry Holt.

Paré, Ambroise. 1582. *Opera omnia.* Parisiis, Iacobus Dv-Pvys.

—— 1594. *Opera chirurgica.* Francofurtus ad Moenum, Ioannis Feyrabend.

Parry, L. A. 1933. *The History of Torture in England.* London, Sampson Low, Marston, pp. v, 1, 2, 178.

Partridge, Eric. 1958. *Origins; A Short Etymological Dictionary of Modern English.* London, Routledge and Kegan Paul.

Paulini, K. F. 1714. *Neu-vermehrte Heylsame Dreck-Apotheke.* . . . Franck-furth am Mayn, Friedrich Knocken, Kap. XXVII.

Payraudeau, B. C. 1828. Note sur le Cuculus hepaticus, de Latham; par M. Mil-let (*Annal. Soc. Linnéenne Paris;* 11ᵉ livrais, mai 1826). *Bull. Sci. nat. Géol., 13,* 241–43.

Peachey, G. C. 1900. Installation of a midwife. *Notes and Queries,* 9th ser., *6,* 177, 438.

—— 1924. Note upon the provision for lying-in women in London up to the middle of the eighteenth century. *Proc. roy. Soc. B, 17,* 72–75.

Pelzeln, August von. 1865. Ueber Farbenabänderungen bei Vögeln. *Verhandl. k.k. zool.-botan. Gesell. Wien, 15,* 911–46.

[Pennant, T.] 1768. *British Zoology.* London, Benjamin White, *1,* 31.

Penny, Frank. 1900. Installation of a midwife. *Notes and Queries,* 9th ser., *6,* 336–37.

Perry, William. [17–?] *The Royal Standard English Dictionary.* . . . Boston, Thomas & Andrews.

—— 1805. *The Synonymous, Etymological, and Pronouncing English Diction-ary.* . . . London, John Walker.

Petrus Hispanus. 1576. *Thesaurum pauperum.* . . . Francof[urtus], Chr. Egen[olff], ff. 73–78.

Pettigrew, T. J. 1844. *On Superstitions Connected with the History and Practice of Medicine and Surgery.* Philadelphia, Ed. Barrington and Geo. D. Haswell, pp. 113–14, 115–16.

Peuckert, W.-E. 1942. *Deutscher Volksglaube des Spätmittelalters.* Stuttgart, Spe-mann, p. 33.

Philips, John. 1923. Folk-lore: Cauls. *Notes and Queries,* 12th ser., *12,* 75.

Photinus. 1621. *Myriobiblion.* . . . Antwerp. Andreas Schott, pp. 1574–75.

Pickin, F. H. 1909. Ancient superstitions that still flourish. *Practitioner, 83,* 848–54.

Pinaeus, I. S. 1563. *De integritatis et corruptionis.* . . . Amstelodami, apud Joan-nem Ravensteinium, pp. 51–52, 103–04.

Bibliography

Piso, Nicolaus. 1580. *De cognoscendis et curandis.* . . . Francofurti, And. Wechelum, *3, 45.*

Pitcairn, Robert. 1833. *Ancient Criminal Trials in Scotland.* . . . Edinburgh, for the Bannatyne Club, *1, 237, 247–53.*

Platerus, Felix. 1666a. *Praxeos medicae opus.* . . . Basileae, Emanuelis König, III, Lib. 2, cap. 1.

—— 1666b. *Centuria posthuma.* . . . Basileae, J. J. Genathi, col. 174.

Plinius Secundus, C. 1601. The Historie of the World. . . . London, Adam Islip. I, Book 8, chap. 42, p. 222; II, Book 28, chap. 11, pp. 326–27.

Ploss, H. 1872. Die Glückshaube und der Nabelschnurrest; Ihre Bedeutung im Volksglauben. *Z. Ethnol., 4,* 186–89.

—— 1884. *Das Kind in Brauch und Sitte der Völker.* Leipzig, Th. Grieben, p. 13.

——, Max Bartels, and Paul Bartels. 1935. *Woman; An Historical, Gynaecological and Anthropological Compendium.* London, Heinemann, *1,* 544, 629–33; *2,* 385, 488–89, 817, 861–64; *3,* 22, 24, 25, 28.

Plutarchus. 1855. *Fragmenta et spuria.* . . . Parisiis, A. F. Didot, vol. XX.

Polwhele, Richard. 1792. *The Idyllia, Epigrams, and Fragments of Theocritus, Bion, and Moschus.* . . . Bath, R. Cruttwell, 2, 29.

Pomet. 1712. *A Compleat History of Drugs.* . . . London, R. Bonwicke, p. 411.

Porta, I. B. 1560. *De miraculis rerum naturalium.* . . . Antverpiae, Christophori Plantini, f. 85.

—— [circa 1910] *La Magie naturelle.* . . . Paris, H. Daragon, chaps. 20, 24, 27.

Preuss, Julius. 1921. *Biblisch-talmudische Medizin.* . . . Berlin, S. Karger, p. 451.

Prick van Wely, F. P. H. 1930. *Engelsch Handwoordenboek.* Den Haag, G. B. van Goor.

Priscianus, Cleopatra, Moschion. 1597. Harmonia gynaeciorum. In: Israelis Spachius, *Gynaeciorum.* . . . Argentinae, Lazari Zetzneri, p. 4.

Puckett, N. N. 1926. *Folk Beliefs of the Southern Negro.* Chapel Hill, University of North Carolina Press, p. 137.

Püschel, E. 1963. Mutter und Kind in der Volksmedizin der Färinseln (Färöer, Føroyar). *Kinderärtzl. Prax., 30,* 123–26.

Quincy, John. 1718. *Pharmacopoeia officinalis.* . . . London, A. Bell, pp. 83, 172.

Rackham, H. 1947. *Pliny; Natural History.* . . . Cambridge, Harvard University Press, VIII, 8; XIX, 9.

Raine, James, ed. 1850. The injunctions and other ecclesiastical proceedings of Richard Barnes, Bishop of Durham, from 1575 to 1587. *Publ. Surtees Soc., 22,* 13–23.

—— 1861. Depositions from the Castle of York. *Publ. Surtees Soc., 40,* xxx, 127.

Raine, James, jun., ed. 1859. The fabric rolls of York Minster. *Publ. Surtees Soc., 35,* 242, 260, 272.

Raines, F. R., ed. 1853. The Derby household books. . . . *Chetham Soc., Remains Histor. Lit., 31,* 153–54.

Ratcliffe, Thomas. 1876. An old Cumbrian custom. *Notes and Queries,* 5th ser., 6, 24.

Ray, John. 1874. *A Collection of English Words not Generally Used.* . . . London, Trübner.

R. C. 1861. Midwives. *Notes and Queries,* 2nd ser., *11,* 59.

Reichelt, Julius. 1692. *Exercitatio de amuletis.* Francofurti & Lipsiae, apud Fridericum Groschuffium, Plate VII.

Reinhard, Felix. 1916–17. Gynäkologie und Geburtshilfe der altägyptischen Papyri. *Sudhoffs Arch. Gesch. Med., 9,* 315–44; *10,* 126–61.

Remy, Nicholas. 1930. *Demonolatry.* London, John Rodker.

Renodaeus, Ioannis. 1631. *De materia medica.* . . . Hanoviae, apud David Aubri., 2, 298, 300.

Renouf, P. le Page. 1873. Note on the medical papyrus of Berlin. *Z. Ägypt. Sprache Alterthumskunde, 11,* 123–25.

Rhazes. *Zehn Bücher an den König Al Mansur.* Lib. V, cap. 69; VI, 27 [cited by Ploss et al., 1935].

Rhodion, Eucharius. [1526] *De partu hominis.* . . . Franc[kfurt], Chr. Egen[olff], cap. 6, f. 25 v.

Ribbeck, Otto. 1894. *P. Vergili Maronis Bucolica et Georgica.* Lipsiae, Teubner, Ecl. XI, lines 23–25.

Ricci, J. V., trans. 1950. *Aetios of Amida.* . . . Philadelphia and Toronto, Blakiston, p. 20.

Riedel, J. G. F. [n.d.] De Sulanezen, hunne gebruiken bij huwelijken, geborte en bij het mutileeren des lichaams. *Bijdr. tot de Taal-, Land- en Volkenkunde van Nederl.-Indie,* 4. Volg. X. D1.3 stuk, 10 [cited by Ploss et al., 1935].

―――― 1886a. *De sluik- en kroesharige Rassen tusschen Selebes en Papua.* s'Gravenhage [cited by Ploss et al., 1935].

―――― 1886b. De Topantunuasu of oorspronkelijke volksstammen van Central-Selebes. *Bijdr. tot de Taal-, Land- en Volkenkunde van Nederl.-Indie,* 5. Volg. I. D1 [cited by Ploss et al., 1935].

Riis, Povl, and Fritz Fuchs. 1960. Antenatal determination of foetal sex in prevention of hereditary diseases. *Lancet, 2,* 180–82.

Ringland, John. 1870. *Annals of Midwifery in Ireland.* . . . Dublin, John Falconer, p. 10.

Robin, P. A. 1932. *Animal Lore in English Literature.* London, John Murray, pp. 83–95, 181–88.

Rocheus, Nicholaus. 1586. De morbis mulierum curandis. . . . In: [Caspar Wolff, ed.] *Gynaeciorum.* . . . Basileae, Conradum Waldkirch, pp. 99–100, 202–03.

Römpp, Hermann. 1946. *Chemisches Zaubertränke.* Stuttgart, Franck, pp. 262–65.

[Rösslin, Eucharius] 1513. *Der Swangern frawen und hebamme[n] roszgarte[n].* [Hagenau, Henricus Gran.] III, 4.

―――― 1540. *The byrthe of mankynde.* . . . London, T. R[aynald], Books I, III.

Rogers, Charles. 1869. *Scotland Social and Domestic.* . . . London, Grampian Club, p. 302.

Rollenhagen, Georgen. 1680. *Warhaffte Lügen von Geistlichen und Natürlichen Dingen.* . . . Wahrenberg, Gottlieb, pp. 22–30.

Rønnike, Folke. 1960. The auxin activity of human serum and urine. *Acta pharmacol. (Kbh.), 16,* 203–12.

Bibliography

───── 1961. *Plantehormoneffekten i menneskets serum og urin.* København, Coster, pp. 114–16.

Ronsseus, Baldvinus. 1594. *De hvmanae vitae primordiis.* . . . Lugduni Batavorum, apud Franciscum Raphelengium, pp. 101–07.

Rorie, David. 1904. The obstetric folk-lore of Fife. *Caledonian med. J.,* n.s., *5,* 177–85.

Rose, H. A. 1905. Muhammadan pregnancy observances in the Punjab. *J. anthrop. Inst. London, 35,* 279–82.

Ross, R. 1891. Forecasting the sex of the child before birth. *Lancet, 2,* 610.

Rubin, S. 1888. *Geschichte des Aberglaubens.* Leipzig, Thiele, p. 149.

Rucker, M. P. 1946. Leaves from a bibliotheca obstetrica. *Bull. Hist. Med., 19,* 177–79.

Rudius, Eustachius. 1595. *De humani corporis affectibus.* . . . Venetiis, apud Robertum Meiettum, Lib. II, cap. 60, p. 192.

Rudkin, E. H. 1936. *Lincolnshire Folklore.* Gainsborough, Beltons, p. 22.

Rueff, Jacob. 1554. *Ein schön lustig Trostbüchle.* . . . Zürych, Christoffel Froschouer, I, cap. 3; III, cap. 3; V, cap. 3, 4, 5; VI, cap. 1.

───── 1580. *De conceptu et generatione hominis.* . . . Francofurti ad Moenum, apud P. Fabricium, V, cap. 5.

───── 1637. *The Expert Midwife.* . . . London, Thomas Alehorn, pp. 86–87.

Rueus, Franciscus. 1566. *De gemmis.* . . . [Lugduni, no pub.], *2,* 32, 39, 45, 62, 64–65.

Ruinus, Carolus. 1603. *Anatomia et medicina equorum noua.* . . . Frankfurt am Mayn, Matthias Becker, *4,* 169.

Ruska, Julius. 1896. *Das Steinbuch aus der Kosmographie der Zakarijâ ibn Muhammed ibn Mahmûd al-Kazwînî.* Heidelberg [cited by Ploss et al., 1935].

R. W. 1905. Palindrome. *Notes and Queries,* 10th ser., *3,* 310.

Ryff, W. H. [1545] *Frawen Rosengarten.* Franckfort, Christian Egenolff, *1,* 16 v., 17 v.–18r.

───── 1571. *Confectbuch unnd Hausz Apoteck.* . . . Franckfurt am Meyn, C. Egenolff, f. 260 r., v.

Sachs, Leo, D. M. Serr, and Mathilde Danon. 1956. Prenatal diagnosis of sex using cells from the amniotic fluid. *Science, 123,* 548.

Saintyves, P. 1936. *Pierres magiques.* . . . Paris, Émile Nourry, pp. 28, 150, 157, 230, 241–44.

Salmon, William. 1678. *Pharmacopoeia Londinensis.* . . . London, Thomas Dawks, pp. 250–51, 406, 411–12.

───── 1703. *Collectanea medica.* . . . London, John Taylor, I, chap. 8; II, chap. 25.

Savonarola, I. M. 1560. *Practica maior.* . . . Venetiis, apud Vincentium Valgrisium, Tract. VI, cap. 21.

───── 1561. *Practica canonica de febribus.* . . . Venetiis, apud Vincentium Valgrisium, vol. 98.

Scheftelowitz, Isidor. 1913. Tierorakel im altjüdischen Volksglauben. *Z. Ver. Volkskunde, 23,* 383–90.

Schenk, P. V. 1879. Relation of foetal heart-beat to sex. *St. Louis Courier Med.*, *2*, 117–21.

Schindler, H. B. 1858. *Der Aberglaube des Mittelalters*. Breslau [cited by Holzinger, 1883].

Schneider, J. G. 1788–89. [Notes appended to his edition of: Frederick II of Hohenstaufen, *De arte venandi cum avibus*. Cited by Butter, 1821.]

Schoeller, Walter, and Hans Goebel. 1931. Die Wirkung des Follikelhormons auf Pflanzen. *Biochem. Z.*, *240*, 1–11.

Schroder, John. 1669. *The Compleat Chymical Dispensatory*. . . . London, John Darby, pp. 158–61, 169–78.

Schulenberg, W. von. 1881. Formel "Sator arepo." *Z. Ethnol.*, *30* (suppl.), 85–86.

Schultz, Simon. 1687. De ovo gallinaceo serpentifero. In: Theophilus Bonetus, *Medicina septentrionalis collatitia*. Geneva, Leonardus Chovët, *2*, 976–79, app. to cap. 7.

Schulz, Hugo, ed. 1897. *Das Buch der Natur von Conrad von Megenberg*. . . . Greifswald, Julius Abel, pp. 138, 328–83.

Schurigius, Martinus. 1731. *Syllepsilogia historico-medica*. . . . Dresdae & Lipsiae, B. C. Hekelii, p. 376.

Schwarz, Paul. 1881. Sator arepo Formel. *Z. Ethnol.*, *30* (suppl.), 131–32.

Schwenckfelt, Casparus. 1600. *Stirpium & fossilium Silesiae*. . . . Lipsiae, Davidis Alberti, pp. 208, 361–62.

—— 1603. *Theriotropheum Silesiae* . . . Lignicii, Davidis Alberti, p. 222.

Scotus, Michaelis. 1508. *De procreatione et hominis phisionomia*. . . . Venetiis, Melchioris Sessa.

—— 1665. *De secretis naturae*. Amstelodami, apud Ioannem Ravensteinium, pp. 245–48.

—— 1930. *The Discoverie of Witchcraft*. . . . [No place], John Rodker. Book II, chap. 9; Book III, chaps. 1, 3; Book X, chap. 8; Book XVI, chap. 9.

Sébillot, Paul. 1906. *Le Folk-lore de France*. Paris, E. Guilmoto, *1*, 160; *2*, 242; *3*, 200, 268.

Seligmann, S. 1910. *Der böse Blick und Verwandtes*. . . . Berlin, Hermann Barsdorf, *1*, 141–49, 360; *2*, 30, 131.

—— 1914. Die Satorformel. *Hess. Blätt. Volkskunde*, *13*, 154–83.

—— 1922. *Die Zauberkraft des Auges und das Berufen*. Hamburg, L. Friederichsen, pp. 184–93, 265.

—— 1927. *Die magischen Heil- und Schutzmittel aus der unbelebten Natur*. . . . Stuttgart, Strecker und Schröder, pp. 215–17, 261–65.

Serapio, Ioannis. 1552. *De simplicium medicamentorum*. . . . Venetiis, apud Andream Arrivabenium, f. 140.

Seyfarth, Carly. 1913. *Aberglaube und Zauberei in der Volksmedizin Sachsens*. . . . Leipzig, Wilhelm Heims, pp. 142, 144, 145.

Shadwell, Thomas. 1691. *The Lancashire Witches*. . . . London, R. Clavell, Preface; Act I, pp. 9, 32, 33, 47.

Sharp, Jane. 1671. *The Midwives Book*. . . . London, Simon Miller, pp. 104–05, 156, 180–86, 188, 190, 198, 208, 224–25.

Sharpe, C. K. 1884. *A Historical Account of the Belief in Witchcraft in Scotland*. London, Hamilton, Adams.

Shettles, L. B. 1956. Sex of infant in relation to nuclear morphology of cells in human amniotic fluid. *Fed. Proc., 15,* 170.

Shipley, J. T. 1945. *Dictionary of Word Origins.* New York, Philosophical Library.

Skeat, W. W. 1910. *An Etymological Dictionary of the English Language.* Oxford, Clarendon Press.

———— 1914. *A Glossary of Tudor and Stuart Words.* . . . Oxford, Clarendon Press.

———— 1924. *The Complete Works of Geoffrey Chaucer.* . . . Oxford, Clarendon Press. W. of B. Prologue, lines 673–77.

———— and C. O. Blagden. 1906. *Pagan Races of the Malay Peninsula.* London, Macmillan, *2,* 23.

Sind, J. B. von. 1770. *Vollständiger Unterricht in den Wissenschaften eines Stallmeisters.* Göttingen und Gotha [cited by Thieke, 1911].

Smith, B. E., ed. 1911. *The Century Dictionary.* . . . New York, Century.

Smith, J. A. 1859. Notices of the hen pheasant assuming the male plumage, with an exhibition of the diseased ovaries. *Proc. roy. phys. Soc. Edinb., 2,* 58–59.

———— 1866. Ornithological notes. 1. *Buteo lagolopus* (Rough-legged Buzzard); 2. *Tetrao urogallus* (Capercailzie, female assuming male plumage); 3. *Saxicola oenanthe* (Wheat-ear). *Proc. roy. phys. Soc. Edinb., 3,* 408–09.

Smith, Johannis, ed. 1722. *Historiae ecclesiasticae gentis Anglorum.* . . . Cantabrigiae, Typis Academicis, Appendix, XV.

Smith, William, ed. 1849. *Dictionary of Greek and Roman Biography and Mythology.* Boston, Little, Brown, *1,* 996–97.

Smoll, Godfrid. 1610. *Manuale rerum admirabilium et abstrusarum.* . . . Hamburgi, Frobenianum, pp. 124–26.

Snell, F. J. 1911. *The Customs of Old England.* London, Methuen, pp. 127–28.

Snell, Otto. 1891. *Hexenprozess und Geistesstörung.* München, p. 81 [cited by Lea, 1939].

Solingen, Cornelius. 1693. *Handbuch der Chirurgie* [cited by Aschheim, 1930].

Solinus, G. J. 1554. *Polyhistor.* Poitiers, Enguilbert Marnes, p. 122.

Sollmann, Torald. 1957. *A Manual of Pharmacology.* . . . Philadelphia, Saunders, pp. 28, 674.

Spence, Lewis. 1920. *An Encyclopaedia of Occultism.* London, George Routledge.

Spencer, H. R. 1927. *The History of British Midwifery from 1650 to 1800.* London, John Bale, Sons, & Danielsson, pp. ii–iv.

Spigelius, Adrianus. 1626. *De formato foetu.* Patauij, Io. Bap. de Martinis & Liuiu Pasquatu, pp. 10–11.

Spindler, Paul. 1691. *Observationum medicinalium centuria.* . . . Francofurti ad Moenum, Philippum Fievetum, obs. LXV.

Stadler, Hermann. 1916. *Albertus Magnus De animalibus.* . . . Münster, Aschendorff, Lib. VII, XXII, XXIII, XXV.

Standlee, M. W. 1959. *The Great Pulse; Japanese Midwifery and Obstetrics Through the Ages.* Rutland, Vt., Charles E. Tuttle, pp. 66–67.

Steele, Robert, ed. 1893. *Mediaeval Lore.* . . . London, Elliot Stock, cap. 16; p. 152.

Stemplinger, Edward. 1925. *Antike und moderne Volksmedizin.* . . . Leipzig, Dieterich, p. 94.

Stölker, Carl. 1875–76. Ornithologische Beobachtungen. *Ber. Thätigkeit St. Gall. naturwiss. Ges.*, pp. 140–64.

Strong, A. B., and D. A. K. Steele. 1874. Joint report of one hundred observations made with a view to the determining of the sex in utero. *Med. Examiner, (Chicago)*, *15*, 385–91.

Strype, John. 1822. *Ecclesiastical Memorials.* . . . Oxford, Clarendon Press, *1*, 390–91.

———— 1824. *Annals of the Reformation.* . . . Oxford, Clarendon Press, *1*, 242–43.

Sudhoff, Karl. 1916. Ein Fruchtbarkeitsregimen für Margaretha, Markgräfin von Brandenburg. *Sudhoffs Arch. Gesch. Med.*, *9*, 356–59.

Sue, [P.] 1779. *Essais historiques, littéraires et critiques, sur l'art des accouchmens* Paris, Jean-François Bastien, *1*, 205, 234–35.

Suetonius Tranquillus, Gaius. 1930. Gaius Caligula. In: *Lives of the Caesars.* London, Heinemann, Lib. IV, sect. 50.

Summers, Montague, trans. 1928. *Malleus maleficarum.* . . . [No place], John Rodker, pp. 66, 99–101, 140–41, 268–69.

Sundevall, C. J. 1845. Sterila hönor (Turr) af Orre och Höns. *Öfver. k. vetensk. akadem. Förhand*, pp. 130–31 [cited by Brandt, 1889].

———— 1854. *Svenska Foglarna.* Stockholm, pp. 245, 249, 275 [cited by Brandt, 1889].

Sutton, J. B. 1885. Diseases of the reproductive organs in frogs, birds, and mammals. *J. Anat. Physiol.*, *19*, 121–43.

Swinhoe, Robert. 1863. The ornithology of Formosa, or Taiwan. *Ibis*, *5*, 198–219, 250–311, 377–435.

Swithin, St. 1905. Palindrome. *Notes and Queries*, 10th ser., *4*, 35.

———— 1915. The caul. *Notes and Queries*, 11th ser., *12*, 239.

Sykes, W. 1886. Child's caul. *Notes and Queries*, 7th ser., *2*, 145.

Sylvius, Jacobus. 1548. *Methodvs medicamenta componendi.* . . . Lugduni, Ioan. Tornaesium & Guielmum Gazeium, *1*, 98–100.

Tait, Lawson. 1878. Enlargement of the thyroid body in pregnancy. *Trans. Edinb. obstet. Soc.*, *4*, 81–95.

Tegetmeier, W. B. 1857. Exhibition of specimens illustrating the differences produced in the hens of the common pheasant and domestic fowl by disease or degeneration of the ovary. *Proc. Zool. Soc. London*, *25*, 81.

Teichmeyerus, H. F. 1731. *Institutiones medicinae legalis, vel forensis.* . . . Ienae, Ioh. Felicis Bielckii, pp. 34–40.

Temesváry, Rudolf. 1900. *Volksbräuche und Aberglauben in der Geburtshilfe und der Pflege Neugebornen in Ungarn.* Leipzig, Th. Grieben, pp. 10, 30–33, 64–65.

Temkin, Owsei, trans. 1956. *Soranus' Gynecology.* Baltimore, Johns Hopkins Press, pp., 7, 44–45, 49 ff.

Thieke, Arthur. 1911. Die Hippomanes des Pferdes. *Anat. Anz.*, *38*, 454–60, 464–86.

Thiers, J.-B. 1741. *Traité des superstitions qui regardent les sacremens.* . . . Paris, Compagnie des Libraires, *1*, 367; *2*, 82.

Bibliography

Thilenius, M. G. 1775. *Kurzer Unterricht für den Hebammen, Schwangeren und Wochnerinnen auf dem Lande.* Cassel, Johann Jacob Cramer.

Thimann, K. V. 1948a. Plant growth hormones. In: Gregory Pincus and K. V. Thimann, eds. *The Hormones.* . . . New York, Academic Press, *1*, 21–22.

—— 1948b. Other plant hormones. In: Ibid., p. 107.

Thiselton Dyer, T. F. 1883. *Folk Lore of Shakespeare.* London, Griffith and Farnam, p. 313.

Thomas, D. L., and L. B. Thomas. 1920. *Kentucky Superstitions.* Princeton, University Press, p. 10.

Thompson, D'A. W. 1910. Historia animalium. In: *The Works of Aristotle.* Oxford, Clarendon Press, *4*, Book IX, 49, 631b.

Thompson, E. M., and W. H. Frere. 1928. *Registrum Matthei Parker, Diocesis Cantuariensis, A.D. 1559–1575.* Oxford, University Press, *2*, 470–72.

Thompson, R. C. 1936. *A Dictionary of Assyrian Chemistry and Geology.* Oxford, Clarendon Press, pp. 104–08.

Thompson, R. L. 1929. *The History of the Devil.* . . . London, Kegan Paul, Trench, Trübner, pp. 142–43, 147.

Thorndike, Lynn. 1923, 1934. *A History of Magic and Experimental Science.* . . . New York, Columbia University Press; New York, Macmillan, *1*, 760, 770–71; *2*, 135, 470; *4*, 398; *8*, 7–10.

—— 1960. De lapidibus. *Ambix, 8,* 6–23.

—— 1963. The pseudo-Galen, "De plantis." *Ambix, 11,* 87–94.

Tichomiroff, A. 1888. Androgynie bei dem Vögeln. *Anat. Anz., 3,* 221–28.

Tiedemann, Friedrich. 1814. Zoologie. In: *Anatomie und Naturgeschichte der Vögel.* Heidelberg, Mohr und Zimmer, *3,* 117–20.

Timbs, John. 1873. *Doctors and Patients.* London, Richard Bentley, *1,* 149.

Tobias, R. 1854. *J. Ornithol. Cabanis,* p. 88 [cited by Stölker, 1875–76].

Topsel, Edward. 1658. *The History of Four-Footed Beasts and Serpents.* . . . London, E. Cotes, pp. 677–78.

Trachtenberg, Joshua. 1939. *Jewish Magic and Superstition.* . . . New York, Behrman, pp. 134, 188–89.

Tremearne, A. J. N. [n.d.] *The Ban of the Bori.* . . . London, Heath, Cranton & Ouseley, p. 100.

—— 1912. Notes on the Kagoro and Other Nigerian Head-Hunters. *J. roy. Anthrop. Inst.,* n.s., *42,* 136–99.

Trevelyan, Marie. 1909. *Folk-Lore and Folk-Stories of Wales.* London, Elliot Stock, p. 265.

Trotula. 1574. *De mulierum passionibus.* . . . Venetiis, Vincentium Valgrisium, cap. 11, 13.

Tsay, Queenie. 1918. Chinese superstitions relating to child-birth. *China med. J. 32,* 533–36.

Tschusi-Schmidhoffen, V. von. 1875. Ornithologische Mittheilungen aus Österreich (1874). *J. Ornithol. Cabanis, 23,* 408.

—— 1886. Androgynie bei Ruticilla phoenicurus. *Z. ges. Ornithol.,* pp. 219–22.

Tuckey, T. P. 1878. The position of the placenta relative to sex of the child. *Med. Press, 25,* 211–12.

Turner, William. 1865. Remarks on the assumption of male plumage by the hen of the domestic fowl. *Proc. roy. phys. Soc. Edinb., 3,* 297–99.

Vairus, Leonardus. 1589. *De fascino.* . . . Venetiis, apud Aldum, Lib. I, 5, 14; Lib. II, 114.

Valentinus, M. B. 1722. *Corpus juris medico-legale.* . . . Francofurti ad Moenum, J. A. Jungii, pp. 120–24.

Valleriola, Franciscus. 1595. *Observationum medicinalium.* . . . Lugduni, apud Franciscum Fabrum, *1,* 85.

Van Andel, M. A. 1910. Dutch folk-medicine. *Janus, 15,* 452–61.

Van Espen, D. Z. B. 1784. *Jus ecclesiasticum.* . . . Venetiis [no pub.] *1,* cap. 5, 299; 2, cap. 5, 17–18.

Van Tienhoven, Ari. 1961. Endocrinology of reproduction in birds. In: W. C. Young, ed., *Sex and Internal Secretions.* Baltimore, Williams & Wilkins, 2, 1111–14.

Varignana, Gulielmus. [1596] *Secreta medicinae.* . . . Basileae, Sebastianum Henricpetri, pp. 197, 198, 200–01.

Varro, M. T. 1934. *De re rustica.* London, Heinemann, II, i, 25; II, v, 17.

Vater, Abrahamus. 1725. *De hippomane.* Inaug.-Diss. Wittembergae [no pub.].

Vega, Christophorus à. 1576. *Liber de arte medendi.* Lugduni, apud Gvlielmvm Rovillivm, Lib. III, cap. 21.

Vergilius Maro, Publius. 1938. *Aeneid.* London, Heinemann, Lib. IV, 509–16.

Vesalius, Andreas. 1543. *De humani corporis fabrica.* . . . Basileae, Ioannem Oporinum, p. 543.

Vigfusson, Gudbrand. 1874. *An Icelandic-English Dictionary.* Oxford, Clarendon Press.

Villiers, Elizabeth. 1927. *Amulette und Talismane und andere geheime Dinge.* Berlin, München, Wien, Drei Masken, pp. 94, 155.

Vincent, Eugène. 1915. La Médecine en Chine au XXe siècle. . . . Paris, G. Steinhiel, pp. 89–90.

Vincentius, Burgundus. 1591. *Speculi majoris.* . . . Venetiis, apud Dominicum Nicolinum, Lib. I, cap. 77.

—— 1624. *Opus praeclarum.* . . . Dvaci, Balthazar Bellerum, pp. 503, 506, 1178–79.

Waite, A. E. 1894. *The Hermetic and Alchemical Writings of . . . Paracelsus.* London, James Elliott, 2, 218.

Wallace-James, J. G. 1900. Installation of a midwife. *Notes and Queries,* 9th ser., *6,* 177.

W. and D. 1785. Midwives formerly baptized infants. *Gentleman's Mag., 55,* 939.

Warden, L. C. 1938. *The Life of Blackstone.* Charlottesville, Va., Michie, pp. 377–78.

Warrack, Alexander. 1911. *A Scots Dialect Dictionary.* . . . London, W. & R. Chambers.

Wasicky, Rich., D. Brandner, and C. Hauke. 1933. Beiträge zur Erforschung der Hormonwirkungen. *Biol. Gen., 9,* 331–50.

Bibliography

Wathen, W. H. 1880. Diagnosis of sex, presentation and position of foetus. *Med. surg. Reporter (Philadelphia)*, *42*, 427–29.

Weber, Max. 1890. Über einen Fall von Hermaphroditismus bei Fringilla coelebs. *Zool. Anz.*, *13*, 508–12.

Weckerus, I. I. 1587. *De secretis.* . . . Basileae, Lemno Valdkirchiana, pp. 108, 176.

Wedelius, G. W. 1725. *Propempticon inaugurale de hippomane.* Ienae, I. F. Ritteri.

Wedgwood, Hensleigh. 1872. *A Dictionary of English Etymology.* New York, Macmillan.

Weekley, Ernest. 1921. *An Etymological Dictionary of Modern English.* London, Murray.

Weeks, W. S. 1923. Folk-lore: Cauls. *Notes and Queries*, 12th ser., *12*, 75.

Weissbart, Max. 1905–06. Der Aberglaube im Geschlechtsleben der Frau. *Mutter und Kind*, 172–75, 182–85, 198–200, 212–14, 227–29.

Wentworth, Harold. 1944. *American Dialect Dictionary.* New York, Crowell.

Westropp, T. J. 1911. A folklore survey of County Clare. *Folk-Lore*, *22*, 49–60.

White, Gilbert. 1923. *The Natural History of Selborne.* New York, Dodd, Mead, pp. 421–22.

White, H. G. E., trans. 1919. *Ausonius.* . . . London, Heinemann, p. 76.

Whitmore, B. T. 1899. An obstetrical charm. *Med. Age (Detroit)*, *17*, 97–98.

Widenmannin, Barbara. 1735. *Kurtze, jedoch hinlängliche und gründliche Anweisung Christlicher Hebammen.* . . . Augsburg [cited by Ploss et al., 1935].

Wierus, Ioannes. 1564. *De praestigiis daemonum.* . . . Basileae, Ioannem Oporinum, cap. 20, 39.

——— 1579. *Histoires, disputes et discours.* . . . [no place], Iaques Chovet, Liv. III, cap. 17.

Wieland, O. P., R. S. de Ropp, and J. Avener. 1954. Identity of auxin in normal urine. *Nature*, *173*, 776–77.

Wilde, Lady. 1890. *Ancient Cures, Charms, and Usages of Ireland.* London, Ward and Downey, p. 61.

Wilde, W. R. 1849. A short account of the superstitions and popular practices relating to midwifery, and some of the diseases of women and children, in Ireland. *Mon. J. Med. Sci.*, *101*, 711–26.

Willey, Arthur. 1892. Untersuchung einer hahnenfedrigen Ente. *Ber. Naturforsch. Ges. Freiburg I. B.*, *6*, 57–61.

Williams, Charles. 1901. Installation of a midwife. *Notes and Queries*, 9th ser., *7*, 31–32.

Williams, W. L. 1921. *The Diseases of the Genital Organs of Domestic Animals.* Ithaca, N.Y., the Author, pp. 160–61.

W[illis], R. 1639. *Mount Tabor.* . . . London, R. B. for P. Stephens and C. Meredith, p. 89.

Willughby, Percivall. [c. 1670] "Observations in midwifery." MS, Lib. Roy. Soc. Med., London, f. 1.

Winstedt, R. O. 1925. *Shaman Saiva and Sufi; A Study of the Evolution of Malay Magic.* London, Bombay, Sydney, Constable.

Wirsung, Christophorus. 1568. *Arzney Buch.* . . . Heydelberg, J. Mayer, p. 452.
Witkowski, G.-J. [1887] *Histoire des accouchements chez tous les peuples.* Paris, G. Steinheil, pp. 164–69, 201.
────── [1891] *Accoucheurs et sages-femmes célébrés.* Paris, G. Steinheil, p. 4 et seq.
Wolff, Caspar, ed. 1586. Harmoniae gynaeciorum. In: *Gynaeciorum.* . . . Basileae, Conradum Waldkirch, pp. 2, 9.
Wreszinski, Walter. 1909. *Der grosse medizinische Papyrus des Berliner Museums (Pap. Berl. 3038).* . . . Leipzig, J. C. Hinrichs, pp. v, 106.
Wright, Joseph. 1902. *The English Dialect Dictionary.* . . . London, Henry Frowde.
Wright, R. P. 1964. A Graeco-Egyptian amulet from a Romano-British site at Welwyn, Herts. *Antiq. J., 44,* 143–46.
Wright, Thomas, ed. 1843. *A Contemporary Narrative of the Proceedings Against Dame Alice Kyteler.* . . . London, Camden Soc., pp. i, iii, iv.
────── 1844. On antiquarian excavations and researches in the Middle Ages. *Archaeologia, 30,* 438–57.
────── 1857. *Dictionary of Obsolete and Provincial English.* . . . London, H. G. Bohn.
────── ed. 1863. *Alexandri Neckham De naturis rerum.* . . . London, Longman, Green, Longman, Roberts, and Green, pp. 198, 469.
Wuttke, Adolf. 1900. *Der deutsche Volksaberglaube der Gegenwart.* Berlin, Wiegandt & Grieben, pp. 52, 237, 381.
Wyld, H. C., ed. 1932. *The Universal Dictionary of the English Language.* London, George Routledge.

Yarrell, William. 1827. On the change in the plumage of some hen-pheasants. *Phil. Trans. roy. Soc., B1,* 268–75.
────── 1831. On the assumption of the male plumage by the female of the common Game Fowl. *Proc. Comm. Sci. and Corresp. Zool. Soc. London, 1,* 22.
────── 1843. *A History of British Birds.* London, John Van Voorst, 2, 285–86.
────── 1857. On the influence of the sexual organ in modifying external character. *J. Proc. Linnean Soc. Zool., 1,* 76–82.
Ysambert. 1903, 1905. Les Superstitions médicales en Touraine. *Gaz. méd. centre, Tours, 8,* 41–42; *9,* 69–70; *10,* 3–4, 99–100, 218–19, 305–06.

Zacchia, Paulus. 1674. *Quaestionum medico-legalium.* . . . Lugduni, Germani Nanty, pp. 54–58.
Zahler, Hans. 1898. *Die Krankheit im Volksglauben des Simmenthals.* . . . Inaug.-Diss. Bern, Haller, p. 83.
Zamagna, Bernardus. 1792. *Theocriti, Moschi, et Bionis idyllia omnia.* . . . Parmae. Bodoniansis, III, 1–5.
Zatzmann, V. 1925. Die Sator-Formel und ihre Lösung. *Hess. Blätt. Volkskunde, 24,* 98–105.
Zilboorg, Gregory. 1935. *The Medical Man and the Witch During the Renaissance.* Baltimore, Johns Hopkins Press, pp. 5–10.

Bibliography

Zingerle, Oswald von. 1891. Segen und Heilmittel aus einer Wolfsthurner Handschrift des XV. Jahrhunderts. *Z. Volkskunde, 1,* 172–77, 315–24.

Zollikofer, Clara. 1939a. Zur Wirkung von Oestron und Thyroxin auf ruhende Knospen. *Ber. Dtsch. Botan. Ges., 57,* 67–74.

—— 1939b. Der Einfluss tierischer Hormone auf Pflanzen. *Ber. Schweiz. Botan. Ges., 49,* 427–28.

⤚§ Index